PRESSURE POINTS

*A Spiritual Path To
Conquer Stress*

DON OSGOOD

Other Books By Don Osgood

Available through Hitchhiker Books
Or Distributors below

- Listening For God's Silent
  Language
- Fatherbond
- How To Really Love Your Job

PRESSURE POINTS

*A Spiritual Path
To Conquer Stress*

By Don Osgood

HitchHiker Books
A Division Of
The Career Performance Group, Limited
Stamford, Connecticut

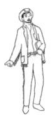

www.hitchhikerbooks.com

FIRST EDITION 1978
FIRST PAPERBACK EDITION 1980
FIRST BALLANTINE BOOKS EDITION 1983
SECOND PRINTING, BALLANTINE BOOKS EDITION JULY, 1985
FIFTH EDITION: HITCHHIKER BOOKS, FEBRUARY, 2002

ISBN 0-9701300-2-3
LIBRARY OF CONGRESS CONTROL NUMBER: 2002090311

Permissions: We acknowledge with appreciation permission to reprint brief passages from:
Toward A Psychology of Being by Abraham Maslow. © 1968. 2nd ed.
  Van Nostrand Reinhold
Childhood and Society by Erik H. Erikson. Rev. ed. © 1963. W. W.
  Norton and Co., Inc.
"Secret of Copying with Stress," *U. S. News & World Report,* March 21, 1977.
"Narcissus Redivivis," *Newsweek*, January 30, 1978

Scripture quotations not otherwise identified are from the King James Version of the Bible.

Printed in the United States of America

NOTE TO THE READER

I don't know if you have ever read a non-fiction book with your "heart" as well as your mind, but I hope you will try with this one. Why? Because you can solve virtually any stress problem-if you will act on the physical, mental and spiritual approaches I discuss in this book. The most complex stress problems can, believe it or not, be identified and healed with surprising freedom.

The way to get the most out of reading *Pressure Points* is to be open to the idea that stress can be handled very well if it is approached honestly and simply. That's not as easy as it sounds, but it can be done. When you reach the stress inventory in Chapter Three, fill in your answers before going on to Part II. Then you will be ready for the excursions into everyday stress problems that I will share with you in the next section. Next, ask yourself as you reach each circumstance and relationship that is explored, "How does this apply to my own life?" If you can, ask for an attitude of personal discernment. Make up your mind even now to talk with someone else about the pressure points in your life that you can identify and understand as you read. The discoveries and approaches in this book should be discussed with others in your family, neighborhood and even place of work. Stress in any part of our lives affects all the other parts.

It is time to bring our Christian and Jewish heritage into our stressful everyday circumstances and relationships. Let your reading of *Pressure Points* be the beginning of a confident attempt to find new freedom in the midst of stress. Read on with your heart. You are about to discover how much our hearts have to do with freedom from stress.

Don Osgood, Stamford, Connecticut

To the people at home and at work who are helping me become more free in the midst of stress

Table of Contents

Part One

Discovering The Sources of Stress for Ourselves

One

That Uncomfortable Feeling Called Stress

We were in a hurry that day. At least I thought we were. A car pulled out right in front of us, and the driver wasn't in a hurry at all. "Why do the slow drivers get in front of me?" I thought. Impatient, I tried to pass, but there was no chance. "What's he doing?" I asked angrily, and my wife, Joan, said, "Maybe God is trying to tell you something, Don."

Maybe so. It was Saturday, and I didn't really need to get anywhere that fast. I had caught the hurry sickness, that uncomfortable feeling of stress from a fast pace of life that carries over into the weekend.

Sometimes you catch stress the way you catch a common cold, by day-to-day exposure. And nobody gets alarmed because everybody knows a little stress won't harm you. Some is actually good for you. But one day you find you have been gripped by the dis-ease of overstress without even knowing when it started. Then you must look for a way out of your illness—for rest from a struggle that is quietly wearing you away.

The University of Washington Medical School came up with 43 life events that make up a stress scale. Seven of the top ten events are directly related to a loss of relationships, such as divorce, death of a spouse, marital separation or retirement. But there is one the scale overlooks: an obedient relationship with God, who won't be pushed, coaxed or manipulated into something that is wrong for us. In the fourth chapter of the letter to the Hebrews an obedient relationship as a way out of the dis-ease of stress is emphasized, so simply that we might easily overlook it: ". . . he that is entered into his rest, he also hath ceased from his own works . . ." (Hebrews 4:10 KJV). This notion of ceasing from personal works was both a message to the Israelites concerning the Sabbath and a reference to the Promised Land. But it is also a God-given prescription for obtaining day-to-day healing from our own stress-struggle.

Take a Look at Yourself

The first step is one of reexamining our egos. Dr. Harry Levinson, the noted psychologist, talks about something called an ego ideal—a bright shiny notion we have of who we might ultimately become. We'll do almost anything to see how big or how good we are, because we want to be able to like ourselves. But there is often a gap between what we are and what we'd like to be, and this gap can cause stress dis-ease—or I'll call it *ego stress*—because our egos are what cause the underlying problem. That's why, even though you may have been a committed Christian, you need to reexamine your way of life.

My own experience with this kind of stress taught me a powerful lesson. I was asked by my company if I would consider an assignment in Japan. It was a great ego builder, but I knew that I might create family problems if I accepted. I had already moved my family to four different cities and after one of these moves my oldest son, then 15, ran away for several days. I should have known that I had no business considering another such move now that another son had reached the critical age of 15. But I let management consider me along with others for six long weeks. All the while I kept saying in my prayers, "I won't try to sell myself, God. I'll just let *them* decide." My wife, Joan, said, "I'm praying for direction for us, Don." And I knew the way she said it that she didn't want to go. My 15-year-old son said flatly, "I don't want to go, Dad!"

At the end of the sixth week the announcement was made that another person had been selected. "It's all right," I said. But it was just two days later that I developed an intestinal disorder that wouldn't go away, and only then did I begin to realize how deep the struggle had been. After four days of discomfort I was awakened in the middle of the night by the same trouble, and with the honesty that exhaustion brings I prayed softly, "I understand now how deeply I have struggled, Lord. Heal me of my sin of preoccupation with *my* wants. Heal my relationship with my family . . . and please heal me of my physical discomfort, too."

I never had to get out of bed that night because my sin was forgiven, and my difficulty instantly vanished along with the tension. I had finally learned a powerful lesson. A person can get so busy gaining a place in life that he risks losing his own family and spiritual relationships.

If your way is to take charge of life without also learning to really let go, or if you are conducting an ego struggle with God, then you are living in *your* kingdom instead of in his way.

The ability to take charge is an important skill in our busy world, and ego is an important part of that. God created us with egos to enable us to achieve. But it's the preoccupation with ourselves that God objects to, because that is what keeps us in bondage to ourselves. Probably 90 percent of our life is spent in thinking about ourselves and in racing after our ego ideal. But God's plan for us when we are overstressed is that we cease from our own works and become occupied again with him. According to an old Spanish proverb, "It is not the burden but the overburden that kills the beast." In other words, it's the normal stress of the day plus the worry over ourselves that harms us. Jesus knew this when he said, "Come unto me, all ye that labor and are heavy laden [overburdened, overstressed, exhausted from the rat race] and I will give you rest" (Matthew 11:28 KJV). It's a way of restful obedience.

Make Up Your Mind

But there is another kind of stress caused by the turmoil of indecision. When I was living in Kansas City, trying to decide which way to turn because of a company reorganization, I was offered a job in Chicago and another in New York. I wanted to stay in Kansas City, but Joan didn't. I thought I was being called into a ministry there with an evangelical organization, but they said, "Both you and your wife must feel the call," and Joan just didn't feel it.

After several weeks of unrest, I consulted a Christian brother who suggested a way to resolve the stress of uncertainty when there is disagreement among the people who are most deeply involved.

"There are three things you must do," he said. "Confess all the sin in your life and clear away anything that stands in the way of a pure relationship with God. Next, explain your problem to him as frankly as you can. Last, believe that he is now working out your answer—not that he will, but that he *is*. Then let it go." That's called abandonment. I had taken the first two steps, but not this third and most important one. When I told God I believed he was working out the answers—in that moment—I found out where I was to go just ten minutes later.

A businessman was late for a speaking engagement in Rochester, Minnesota, and was just leaving Minneapolis, 80 miles away, with no lunch and only an hour and a half before he was to speak. Though he normally drove at 55 miles per hour, he sped down the highway at a breathtaking 85, until a state trooper spotted him. He saw the trooper looking right at him as he raced by, and he prayed, "Lord, you know I need to get to Rochester. Don't let him stop me." But something checked him and he added, "If that's all right with you." Apparently it wasn't all right, because the trooper stopped him and asked where he was going. He said, "To give a lecture on stress." Then, feeling very sheepish, he added, "And I feel very stressed right now."

We don't want to meet people when we've been doing wrong, especially people in authority. But it reduces stress to admit we're wrong. Though it's not fun, it's strangely more freeing to be caught when we're guilty than to carry around the knowledge of guilt. Sooner or later we must come to terms with our guilt or lose the openness that makes a real spiritual relationship possible.

It works the same way with stress caused by self-doubt. A friend of mine began to feel that his company was counting too much on his ability to discover new technical solutions and that he wasn't making the progress he felt he ought to make. His nagging doubts that he couldn't live up to the expectations of others finally landed him in the hospital, until he realized that secure relationships are built on who we are, not on what people want us to be. When a psychiatrist finally asked my friend after a year of counseling, "Why are you so hard on yourself? God loves you," he began to be healed.

If we are still running our lives on the assumption that God expects us to be good we are living a lifestyle of ego stress, however unaware of it we may be. When we realize that God loves us, knowing that we can't be good without him, we are getting closer to freedom. Christ's cure is, in effect, "Don't try harder. Don't even think harder. Instead of going your own way, yield more." He said it in a different way in the Sermon on the Mount: "Consider the lilies." But the more successful we become the harder it is to see the lilies, let alone consider them. When we really consider a lily, we begin to realize that it is beautiful just by being what God wants it to be, without being fretful about what it might become or what it can't become.

If you won't relearn how to trust in our Lord's plan, you may be flirting with an anxiety condition somewhere down the road. Christ had strong feelings about this. "Don't be anxious," he said. When a task is so huge that you can't see the end of it, but you know you must get it done in a month, decide exactly how much you will do today. Don't get sidetracked by what you must have accomplished two weeks from now. This is a practical way of following Christ's statement that we are not to be anxious about tomorrow. Instead of healing your anxiety, Christ wants to heal you of the condition that could lead you there.

Stress Signals

Here are some of the day-to-day stress signals to be aware of:

An unexplained change in your effectiveness. You suddenly realize you are unable to perform satisfactorily in an activity that you used to do well.

Irregular performance. You were highly effective just last week, but this week, for some reason, you can't seem to get anything done.

A pattern of absence. You find youself taking a day off or filling up your time with other "important" things when a certain activity or appointment with someone is coming up.

Cooled relationships. People with whom you used to get along well are not as warm and natural with you as they used to be.

These and other signals indicate that stress may be getting to you and that you should do something about it.

What are some day-to-day causes of preoccupation with ourselves and the resulting faithlessness and disobedience we may have?

Sudden change—whether we bring it about ourselves or whether someone else does. Has life shifted you into a new responsibility that you aren't ready for, or one that calls on your weaknesses instead of your strengths? Have you just moved or are you about to move?

Thwarted ambition. Have you become middle-aged without reaching the life goals you once hoped to achieve, and with little chance you'll ever reach them?

The fear as you grow older that your capabilities are waning. Usually this fear is groundless. Your capabilities change as you mature, but you develop new strengths to offset reduced ability in others.

Personality clashes. These often occur because someone is trying to bend you to their desire for your life—or you are trying to bend someone to your notion of the way they should live. Either way, people don't like to be changed by others, and when the attempt is made, stress occurs. Sometimes it should, such as during the parental guidance years. But disciplining someone in the way of the Lord and controlling or manipulating that person are two entirely different things. Disciplining should happen. Controlling should not—whether you are a minister or a manager or a mother.

Doing something that violates your conscience. It takes maturity and courage to stand up for what you believe, and say to your neighbor or your superior, "This is something I won't do." It may cost you a return invitation or even a job sometime during your life, but it shows a special loyalty and it helps you live with yourself.

Preventive Maintenance

Here are some practical, preventive maintenance steps to help keep you from anxious living—from grabbing back the style of living in your own strength. You should consider these steps only after you have renewed an obedient relationship with God and believe he is doing his work in you. Then you can take some action.

Learn to temporarily set aside your problems. When you're in the middle of a stressful situation, develop the ability to temporarily put it out of your mind. Concentrate on something strikingly different for a predetermined time period, after which you'll return to the problem. Say to yourself, "It's O.K. for me not to be involved in that for the next hour because I can't handle it right now." The advice given in Proverbs 3:5, "Trust in the Lord and lean not unto your own understanding," really represents a faith relationship applied to a specific problem.

Follow an unconventional schedule. Work on your difficult tasks early in the morning when you can do them with none of the distractions that cause stress. Learn to wait prayerfully for the Lord's instructions for the day by following Christ's example of rising very early in the morning to pray.

Write "memos" to God. If you're caught in a stressful situation, scribble out a forceful note explaining your feelings in plain and strong terms. Write down exactly what disturbs you. Name specific persons and actions that bother you. Get your feelings out of your system. Just writing them down often gives you a different perspective, makes the problem more manageable and relieves the stress. Don't tell yourself you don't feel bad when you do. Be honest and tell God the truth. Admit your need and ask him to help you release the things you have written down.

Change your environment. Take 20 minutes off for vigorous jogging, followed by a shower or swim. Or have a leisurely lunch by yourself. Or when stress builds up, walk off your problem outdoors. The important thing is to change your physical environment completely. Sometimes do it more elaborately. For instance, go on a weekend trip with your wife or husband without the children and rediscover the joy and the importance of your relationship. All of these are good times to reestablish your dialogue with the Lord.

Find a model to follow. Think about the humanness of Christ and why he handled far more stress than you, successfully. He could do it not only because he was God, but because he did something as a person. One of the things he did was to get away by himself. He practiced it throughout his adult life.

Find a "special" someone who can help you. Select a person or persons whom you particularly admire, whom you can trust to be honest with you and feel you can turn to for advice on your own problems. (Not necessarily one in authority over you and not someone you expect to bail you out of trouble.) Pick someone with whom you can pray in an open way, or silently. Either way, prayer with a friend who will make you honest with yourself is a special stress reliever. Recognize while you are praying that God is interested in the real source of your concerns. That's one reason why he wants two or more of us agreeing together.

A Place of Rest

The children of Israel failed to enter into their Promised Land because of their disobedience, lack of faith in God, and tendency to trust solely in their own remedies. That truth applies to you and me. Our modern place of rest is as available as the Promised Land was to the Israelites— without years of counseling or personal struggle.

Look closely at verses 9 and 10 of Hebrews 4. They offer the model of rest actually practiced by God. "There remaineth therefore a rest to the people of God. For he that is entered into his rest, he also hath ceased from his own works, *as God did from his.*" That's God's pretested way out of the wilderness of overstress. He replaces stress with rest. When you believe that the teachings of his Son Jesus are commandments to be obeyed, promises to be believed and examples to be used on a daily basis, then you are beginning to reduce the ego struggle that causes stress.

To regain freedom from stress, there are a number of day-to-day principles we can use. But the real solution is in finding how to abandon ourselves to God as enthusiastically as a young child jumps into a pool. The word *enthusiasm* has come to describe our attitude when we enter into some activity, but it originates from the Greek *en* and *theos*, meaning God within. We receive God's inner healing from stress by ceasing from our own lifestyle and literally jumping into his.

Be healed of your own way, whatever it is, by abandoning yourself to God's healing. Obey. Believe. Then you are free to do—without the disease of overstress.

This involves digging down and getting real with ourselves and the people around us. It involves a willingness to look at where stress really comes from and to learn how to get *out* of control, rather than in control. From a secular view this notion makes no sense at all. That's why we will need to look more closely at several views to understand better where stress really comes from.

Two

Where Stress Really Comes From

It was just three weeks before my son's graduation from high school. He had fallen in love with a sixteen-year-old girl who was powerful in more ways than one. She was a good-looking blonde with a sweet smile and a way about her that made my son want to take care of her. "I love her, Dad," he said. "She doesn't have much. I want to help her." Unfortunately, he soon began to come home very late at night. When I told him he couldn't stay out late, especially with just three weeks to go before final exams, he showed me that he could and left home.

I knew I couldn't hold him at home at eighteen when he had already made up his mind to live somewhere else. He came home for his things one night and was down in the garage, getting his tools together. He didn't look up when I came in. In my emptiness I didn't know what to say.

"I hope you'll finish school, son," I said. He didn't answer.

"You'll have a place here if you want to come home."

I looked at him closely, not knowing what his reaction would be, and I reached out to him.

"I love you, son."

I was experiencing the stress of a lost relationship.

What's the cause of stress? Where does it come from? It comes from economic crises, energy shortages, and deeper things, like uneasy relationships—literally from everywhere, because one person's stress is another person's challenge.

If we really want to know where stress comes from we must be willing to become open to the subject in a personal way, because stress is a very personal matter. We can deny that it exists. We can participate in some form of meditation or exercise or diet control, and get help from all of these. Or we can go even beyond this by seeking discernment of stress and deal with it on a deeper level. But we must not deny that we have stress. I know about denial because I have done it, even as a practicing Christian. Denial doesn't resolve stressful living.

It's not someone else's stress we are talking about. It's concern about our own stress that's important. Why else has the word, "relax" become so often used in our daily talk? The biblical observation by Jeremiah that people will cry for peace yet there is no peace applies today, and it doesn't necessarily mean that we are seeking merely the absence of war. In peace time we still seek peace, because we are living stressful lives. We can't just wish away or meditate away our stress. Some people are supposedly meditating stress away and losing their families while doing it.

Discovery is an important step, as long as it leads us to decision. Take a look at the complete list of the stress causes that two doctors developed. If we look at the first 10 causes, as mentioned in chapter one, we can draw our own conclusion about the impact of loss of relationship. Most of us have not experienced the hardship of this much stress in the past year or so, but whatever our circumstances have been it is appropriate to face them squarely with some idea of what to do about them.

RANK	EVENT
1	Death of spouse
2	Divorce
3	Marital separation
4	Jail term
5	Death of close family member
6	Personal injury or illness
7	Marriage
8	Fired from work
9	Marital reconciliation
10	Retirement
11	Change in family member's health
12	Pregnancy
13	Sex difficulties
14	Addition to family
15	Business readjustment
16	Change in financial status
17	Death of close friend
18	Change to different line of work
19	Change in number of marital arguments
20	Mortgage or loan over $10,000
21	Foreclosure of mortgage or loan
22	Change in work responsibilities
23	Son or daughter leaving home
24	Trouble with in-laws
25	Outstanding personal achievement
26	Spouse begins or stops work
27	Starting or finishing school
28	Change in living conditions
29	Revision of personal habits
30	Trouble with boss
31	Change in work hours, conditions
32	Change in residence
33	Change in schools
34	Change in recreational habits
35	Change in church activities
36	Change in social activities
37	Mortgage or loan under $10,000
38	Change in sleeping habits
39	Change in number of family gatherings
40	Change in eating habits
41	Vacation
42	Christmas season
43	Minor violation of the law

Drs. Holmes and Rahe state that future illness will occur more frequently where we experience high levels of stress. But with each of these causes of stress, however cutting or harmful, there is an active, confident approach to every one of these life experiences that can help us.

There are at least five layers to deal with in managing stress. We can deal with these layers one at a time and get a measure of freedom or we can go right to the center of the issue, where stress really comes from. But we must remember that we won't ever be totally released from stress itself. We need to be clear about that, because some stress is woven into life itself for a purpose. It's stress *reaction* that we need to consider as well. It's the overbearing or accumulated stress to be concerned about.

The five layers we will deal with can be seen more clearly in this drawing.

FIVE LAYERS IN MANAGING STRESS

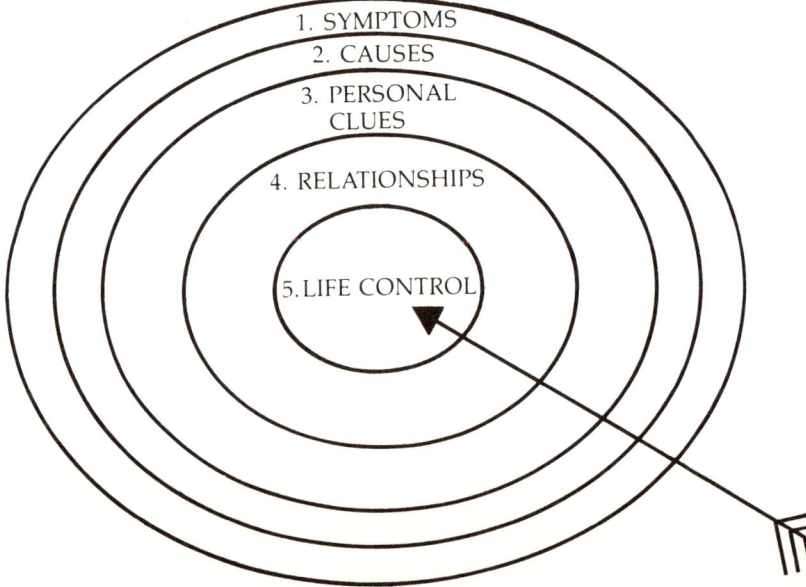

1. SYMPTOMS
2. CAUSES
3. PERSONAL CLUES
4. RELATIONSHIPS
5. LIFE CONTROL

Each layer can be expressed in terms of what to do about it: (1) Watch the symptoms. Even these can add to our stress. (2) Examine the causes. There is usually a cause that is separate from the symptom. (3) Consider some clues. But be aware that an underlying condition is the key. (4) Analyze the impact of others. There is always a force-field of personal relationships going on and our relationships cause much of our stress. (5) Resolve the issue of life-control. This is where much of our basic stress comes from.

Why talk about layers of stress? Because often we know that something in our lives isn't as it should be, but we don't know where to start setting things right. So while we wait for something to come along that will help, we deal with stress in a shallow way. Perhaps we're like Henry, a church member who always responded to the visiting minister's call during the annual spring revival. When the invitation was given to come forward for healing, Henry would start down the aisle from the back of the church, loudly imploring, "Fill me full, Lord, fill me full." Again as he neared the front he would repeat, "Fill me full, Lord, fill me full." When Henry did this one spring the pastor overheard a member of the congregation say quietly, "Don't do it, Lord. He leaks."

All of us leak. We want to do right; we want to put the pressures of life into the right perspective, but we forget how, and we wait for some meeting or method before dealing with life. Henry didn't need to wait for the spring revival for healing. We, like Henry, need to realize that God wants to deal with our stresses *where we are, when they happen.* But God has difficulty filling us up when we aren't empty of ourselves. We need to stop telling God how to cure us and simply open up ourselves for his healing—in his way.

Looking at the layers of stress, the first two were covered briefly in chapter one. Now let's take a look at the third step. Under the third layer, there are personal and family clues that we can look for in four specific relationships and four definite areas of our life. The four relationships are: wife or husband, children, parents and self. The four areas are: finances, health, pace of life and career. There are others concerning the future that we will deal with later. Each one of these immediate areas may be a rock under which our specific stress is hiding. If we can turn over the rocks we stand a better chance of being free of the disease of stress.

The following questions may help you turn over a rock or two. In the column on the right side circle the answer you feel applies to you. If you would rather not show your answers in this book you can list them on a separate sheet by putting the question numbers down the left side, from one to twenty-five. What you are about to do is inventory your own marriage, family and personal circumstances to find some additional clues to where stress may be coming from.

MARRIAGE, FAMILY AND PERSONAL
STRESS INVENTORY

Consider your circumstances over the past few months and put a circle around the answer that applies to you.

SPOUSE: **Y   Z**
  1. Has your wife or husband been trying to   No   Yes
     change your attitude or way of life
     recently, against your wishes?

2.	Do you feel your wife or husband loves you more than (or about as much as) in the first year of your marriage?	Yes	No
3.	Have your own or your spouse's beliefs regarding sexual faithfulness changed in the recent past?	No	Yes

CHILDREN:

4.	Do you and your wife or husband basically agree on the way to bring up your children (or on the way they were brought up)?	Yes	No
5.	Have you had strong disagreements recently with your wife or husband over one or more of your children (regardless of their age)?	No	Yes
6.	Have one or more of your children been showing a rebellious or unresponsive attitude recently, or doing things that are against your specific wishes or instructions for them?	No	Yes

PARENTS — RELATIVES:

7.	Do your own or your spouse's parents or relatives give you freedom to run your own household without interfering in what you believe to be right?	Yes	No
8.	Do your parents or relatives maintain strong disapproval of your way of life (your values) as an individual, even though there is no active interference?	No	Yes
9.	Do your or your spouse's parents often try to tell you what to do, even concerning insignificant matters?	No	Yes

SELF:

10.	Do you hide your feelings of disagreement, frustration or anger with your wife, husband or others and not reveal them?	No	Yes

11. Have you been interested as much in others—your family or friends—lately, as much as you have been interested in yourself, your career or your own activities?	Yes	No
12. Do you have someone you can confide in, who really listens to your concerns and cares for your well-being?	Yes	No

FINANCES:

13. Do you have disagreements over who should handle family finances or how they should be handled?	No	Yes
14. Do you find that bills or credit accounts are piling up and you are not quite sure whether there will be money enough to pay them on time?	No	Yes
15. Are either your savings or your job security eroding to the point that it bothers either you or your spouse?	No	Yes

HEALTH:

16. Is there an unexplained physical change that you have noticed in yourself that has been on your mind?	No	Yes
17. Have you discovered, after medical advice or assistance, that there is something wrong with you physically that wasn't wrong a few months ago?	No	Yes
18. Are you about as capable of physical recreation, strenuous work or exercise as you were a few months or a year ago?	Yes	No

PACE OF LIFE:

19. Do you have time to do most of the things you need to do to keep your personal and family responsibilities in order?	Yes	No
20. Are there a number of things you have been wanting to do for some time now that you never seem to get around to do?	No	Yes

21. Are work, social or community commitments   No   Yes
crowding out your time for the family
relationships that you want to have?

CAREER:
22. In your opinion, are you viewed as   Yes   No
favorably in your organization as
you were a year or so ago?
23. Do you enjoy the day-to-day work in   Yes   No
your present job as much as you have
enjoyed your work in previous jobs?
24. Is your career or your spouse's   No   Yes
career causing family difficulties
that are a source of disagreement?

PERSONAL ACCEPTANCE:
25. Except for a few changes, perhaps,   Yes   No
are you basically satisfied with and
accepting of yourself?

SCORING INSTRUCTIONS:
Add the number of Y responses and Z responses for each of the
areas covered:

		Y	Z
1.	Spouse		
2.	Children		
3.	Parents — Relatives		
4.	Self		
5.	Finances		
6.	Health		
7.	Pace of Life		
8.	Career		
9.	Personal Acceptance		
	TOTAL		

If your Z responses add up to 12 or more they suggest that marriage, family or personal circumstances may be presenting an overall problem warranting your attention. If you have a greater number of Y responses than Z responses, it is likely that you have less overall stress, although a high number of Z responses in any one category may warrant your attention. If one or more areas do not apply to your circumstances, disregard them. Use 11 as your "attention" number if only seven areas apply. Use 10 if only six areas apply, and so on.

Now that you have looked over the questions and have completed your self-score you might feel like Vincent, who took a similar inventory during a weekend retreat. "I didn't have any stress when I came," he said. "But now I do." He was having a little fun with me about it and I hope you will, too, even though you may be saying to yourself quite sincerely, "I see an area or two that I would like to pay some attention to, but *now* what do I do?" Or you may find no appreciable sign of stress at all. There may be denial of stress. Or there may be other areas of stress that are not included in this inventory. But with *any* of these outcomes it helps to discuss your inventory with your wife, husband, or a person you trust. Your own or a neighboring pastor can be of real help here as well. Recognizing and discussing different perceptions about stressful living could temporarily increase stress. But agreement on areas that can be changed can reduce it—and make your relationship open and more fruitful.

The most critical stress doesn't happen at work. It happens in our personal lives, in our homes and in our relationships. When I added up my responses in the "z" column I had a fairly low score of 10, but I found that children, finances, pace of life and self were areas that needed my attention.

One group of married men that completed a marriage, family and personal stress inventory ranged from age 30 or so to the early 60's and their responses in the "z" column were higher in the same areas as mine: children, finances, pace of life and self. For others, the responses were different and they varied with circumstances over the past several months. In general, relationships with wife or husband are an area of high stress as well.

But there are other areas. Worry over the future is one. When the economy threatens our home or our standard of living, we worry. When we fly in a plane we worry. Have you ever noticed how much a stranger will tell you on a plane? It's a good way to handle stress. At least it's a lot less expensive than going to a psychiatrist! Travelers on buses and trains often will tell you things about their past that they wouldn't say if they knew you. But in a plane there seems to be a special desire to talk. Perhaps when the future seems a little less certain we talk more about who we really are, where we are going and where we've been. And it's not just travel schedules. When I sat next to a successful businessman on a rough flight to Atlanta he told me about the way he had made his money through kickbacks and racketeering in the bowling industry. He mentioned his son who had run away, his wife who had been institutionalized and his practice of wearing a gun for personal protection from the organization. Stress in one area had made its impact in several others, as it usually does, and now guilt had entered in. He looked at me from his window seat and said, "I don't like to fly." We talked then about the future and about God.

These two areas, the future and God, aren't often brought up in discussions about stress, but they are important areas. "Where am I heading?" is one of the more profound questions in career or home life for anyone who hasn't looked at all of life squarely. When that question is raised with a group of career people there is a lot of interest in how to answer it. But whenever we think of the future the past usually comes up. We stuff the past back down quickly or we look at it without guilt depending on how the past has been dealt with. The future and the past bring us into a square look at God, even if only fleetingly on a plane.

At our own time and place we are often willing to talk about these things *because we know deep down inside that stress is relieved when we talk to someone,* whether or not the person has words of advice. It helps to talk with a real friend whom we can trust. Talking to a trusted friend who can help us open up is even more fruitful. And that brings us to a consideration of why God wants us to talk to him. If that is God's desire, what keeps him out of our lives? If there are barriers, what are they?

Many of us go through a part of our lives holding onto a little red wagon of things we have done that are not settled up. These may include unresolved relationships at home or old hurts at the hand of someone, or things we have done that we wish we had not done. And there are things we haven't done that we now wish we had. If we don't settle these things we trail them around with us, buried way down in the bottom of the wagon. The ones that are in the bottom are often the ones we don't want to see anymore, but they are there and they cause extra effort in life because of the extra weight we are pulling. Pulled long enough, the weight in the wagon begins to tire us out, sap our energy and even make us susceptible to illness.

Take the case of Karen, who has been pulling a loaded wagon around for years. After a while she started developing a series of unexplained illnesses. Later on she experienced a series of accidents. Now the pattern of the past is clear. Karen is illness prone, accident prone, and worry prone. She is an unhappy Christian and doesn't even know it. But her past is finding her out. The statement that we are to be sure our sins will find us out is literally a prescription for freedom from an unhappy life. If only we could tip our wagon over, empty it and push it over a cliff. What we need to pray is not, "Fill me full, Lord," but "Empty me, Lord, so you can fill me full."

The basic issue in a stressful life is wrapped up in the question, "Who's in charge here?" If the answer is, "Me," then basic stressful living is present. One of the most profound truths about stress is found in the realization that outside of the Spirit of God we become tense. In his Spirit we are relaxed. His gift to stressful people is the freedom to be honest with ourselves. We literally don't need to cover up our past or even solve marriage, child or parental problems by ourselves. We can explain to him everything we have done, didn't do, or don't know how to do, *without punishment*. Punishment is something we have already levied upon ourselves. It's almost as though God is saying to us, "Let me hear your problems. But don't try to blame anyone else for them. And don't try to kid me, because I know who you are and where you are heading and how you can get freedom from guilt."

This is the beginning of a relationship based upon reality, not denial. When we realize how capable he is to heal us we no longer have difficulty over who's in charge. We find it quite natural to say, "I don't want to be in charge. I want you in charge." This relationship allows us to drop the handle of our red wagon so we can really embrace God. And that is possible. That is what Christ was talking about. While Christ cured dis-ease he repeatedly showed that the solution was to heal the patient. In effect he was saying, "I want you to realize that you are a patient. You need some help. And I can help you."

There is freedom in knowing we are needy, rather than kidding ourselves that we are self-sufficient. This freedom to be weak—to drop unreality—brings a deeper relationship that we get *without trying to figure it out*. Free hearts communicate without even knowing how!

I saw this all the more as I became willing to look at all my relationships and areas of life and *not* try to solve them by myself! When I invited the real physician to enter into a deeper level he put his finger on specific areas that needed my attention. When I agreed to his probing into these hidden areas, he did the healing. I began to look more closely at Joan and found a new relationship that I couldn't have produced and had not dreamed would ever exist.

Now you and I are ready to deal more thoroughly with each of the four relationships and circumstances in the marriage, family, and personal stress inventory earlier in this chapter. In Part Two I invite you to look deeper into the pressure points that we have just begun to look at. Now you can look at the actual struggles of others who have faced these four relationships and circumstances. In a sense we will do this together because I'm going to try to

hold nothing back, and you can look at your own circumstances and relationships at the same time. Prayerfully and confidently, we are going to experience new
healing insights together, as you compare your own experiences with mine and with others. And we will deal
with pressure points that are *common* to us in our everyday lives.

Now, in the privacy and intimacy of Part Two I invite
you to take a look in the mirror with me and learn how to
be more free.

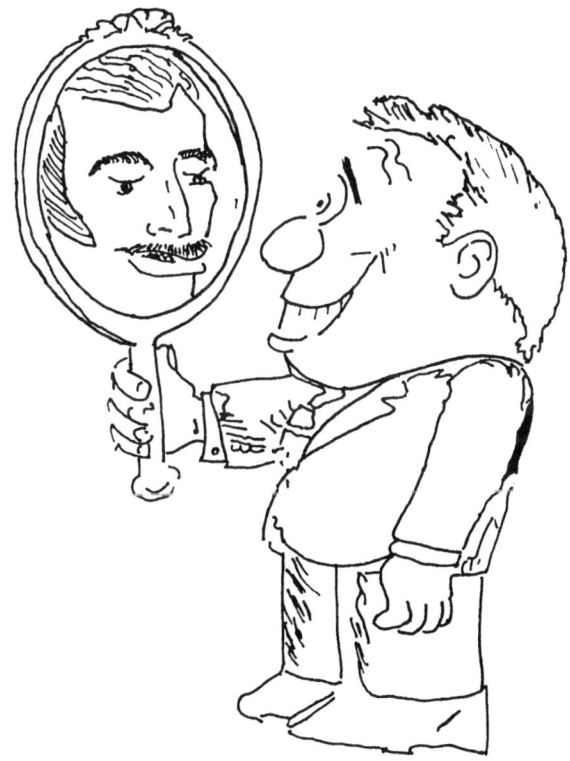

Part Two

*Dealing With Pressure
Points In Our Lives*

Three

Letting Your Cinderella Grow

It had become more and more apparent that my wife, Joanie, did not want to be called Joanie any more. But she thoughtfully didn't require me to change overnight and call her Joan the next morning. That would have been hard to do after 23 years of a special relationship we had both developed. Still there was something unequal about my being called Don, as though only I were grown, and her being called Joanie, as though she were not. But that thought had not occurred to either of us. What had occurred was one of those unquestioning marriages where things seemed to go right from the beginning. Why raise questions when things are going right, or when you think they are?

But sometimes marriages start going wrong very quietly and often long before they fall apart. They dry up before they split. One reason even good marriages fall apart is that unequal relationships develop over the years, and this causes marital stress. Sometimes open discord follows, but other times it is buried or stuffed. Stressful marriage isn't always recognized until one day dawns and the person realizes that love is gone. It's hard to tell when love leaves. In the beginning a man falls in love with a woman, partly because she needs him and believes in him. When she loves him and forsakes everyone else in the world for him, he begins to believe more in *himself* while he learns to love her. So the beginning years of marriage are often a little like the Cinderella story, and that's the way it was with us.

There's a bit of Cinderella and Prince Charming in many marriages. Sometimes it lasts for six months, sometimes for years. But when a woman doesn't want to be Cinderella anymore, it forces a man to stop acting the role of Prince Charming whether he wants to stop or not. Or it causes him to find another Cinderella so he can continue the role.

It works the same way the other way around. When a husband wants to stop being the kind of person he was when he first married, there isn't much choice for a wife who still wants to keep the marriage going. She has to adjust and hope for the best or find another Prince Charming.

Often it isn't anyone else a husband or wife is interested in. Sometimes a person falls in love with his or her career. It's not that a person means to, or that he even knows that he is in love with it. From a career person's point of view, it's necessary to establish a reputation, and that means competing for the assignments that open the doors to more important positions. Bringing work home is a necessary part of a career to an aspiring person, but to the marriage partner who isn't working it's an intrusion on their time together. Over the years sustained success gives additional rewards but requires more time, so that one day without even dreaming that it is happening, a person falls in love with his job. At least it consumes his devotion.

Success itself can change marriage, because it changes the person. It often makes a person self-centered, however interesting or charming he or she is while becoming successful. The wife of a successful doctor expressed her feelings this way: "If I hear one more person glorifying my husband I think I'll scream!"

But success reactions like this aren't confined to doctors or their wives. One happily married man opened a restaurant that became an immediate success, so he expanded it and poured enough money, time and devotion into it that after awhile he couldn't stay away from it. When he and his wife realized what this was doing to their lives they began to counteract the mounting marital stress by closing the restaurant down on certain holidays and going far enough away that he couldn't go in to check on things. This same devotion to achievement can happen in any walk of life, whether it's the ministry or mechanics or medicine. One question married people need to face when they get caught up in other loves like this is: "What's important to me right now, at this point in my life?" And close behind that question is a second: "Who's important to me right now?"

With Joan and me this problem of priorities came to light after years of career success that included speaking engagements around the country. We decided to go on a weekend retreat with other couples from our church and I found myself sitting with a small group of people in open discussion. The leader looked at me after a few minutes of discussion and said, "Mr. Osgood, you don't love your wife." "What do you mean?" I asked, annoyed at her gross error in judgment. "I married Joanie when she was 17. I married her in the Catskill mountains while she was finishing up her final week of senior exams in high school. We've been happily married ever since, and it's been 22 years of pure joy with Joanie. I love her." With that I felt I had settled the issue, but the discussion leader came right back at me.

"You don't love your wife. She's just a part of your arm. You have *acquired* her over the years and now she's just a possession of yours." Then she looked at me closely and asked, "Why do you call her Joanie?"

Later that night I began to see what the discussion leader was talking about. When Joan and I were together this time in another discussion group, the discussion leader asked Joan a question. Joan looked to me for help and then answered in a high pitched voice that sounded like a 17-year-old. The discussion leader looked at me and said, "Do you realize you have frozen your wife at 17?"

I hadn't realized that, nor had Joan. What had been happening in the more recent years of our marriage was a takeover that was slowly squeezing Joan's ego into a corner. My success was costing her something and neither she nor I knew it. Later that night Joan and I had one of the most painful discussions I can remember. We went for a walk to try and put some of the pieces of the day together, and as we were returning to the retreat house she said, "Don, I'm afraid." And she looked up at me with tears running down her face. I looked at her, wishing I could help. "Afraid of what, Joanie?" I asked.

"I'm afraid to find out who I really am. They told me today I've been idolizing you and burying me."

It took many months to work out a new relationship between us. But without the willingness to work at it our marriage might have eroded into a superficial, resigned acceptance of each other without the vibrancy we had first known. My priorities had become mixed up.

Here's a way to check up on your priorities and start a mutual exploration with your mariage partner on ways to reduce marital stress and some of the seeds of potential discord. List ten things that are the most important to you right now, considering all the worlds in which you live. Put them down as they come to mind without attempting to rank them. Include career, family, spiritual and leisure interests. Then put a number beside each one that shows the way you really rank it compared to the others. Put a one by the most important one and a two by the next one and so on until you have a number for all ten items. Don't allow yourself any ties. Then ask your wife or husband to put down ten things that she or he feels are most important right now, ranking them from one to ten in the same manner you have already done for yourself. Then show each other your lists and talk about them. Chances are you will be talking for the rest of the night. Your awareness of priorities and your partner's perception may be totally different, or different enough that you will want to talk them over.

Here's another way to look at what's important: Draw a big circle on a piece of paper and write above it, "This is a typical day (or week) in my life." Then divide the circle up into pieces of pie and make each piece the right size for the amount of time or waking hours you spend for each of the ten important things in your life that you have listed. Here are two examples of the way a circle might look according to Boston College's Dr. Margaret Gorman. After you have looked them over, try your own circle, then show it to your wife or husband.

I drew one of these circles showing my priorities and put it on a blackboard during a discussion at our church one night. Everybody seemed to appreciate how well I had organized my priorities, except for one person in the group, and I found out who that was on my way home. Joan said, "Your circle was wrong." Then she looked at me closely. "How much time do you really spend with our children?" I thought for a moment, then Joan helped my thoughts a bit further. "How much time are you spending with your last son, Trevor? Remember him?" It was one of those moments of truth you get when someone else looks at your life and informs you what it looks like from another vantage point.

Often I find people who look at a circle like this and realize it's not always the amount of time they spend on a certain priority or relationship but the *quality* of time. Sometimes an hour of real sharing is worth eight hours of superficial time, but this can be a way to rationalize, too. Letting someone else look at the circle of your priorities can be a fruitful time, if an honest but loving discussion reveals that something needs to be adjusted.

One couple—we'll call them Ivan and Maureen—had allowed their marriage to become a stressful relationship on a very conscious level. I received a call from Ivan one day. "I need your prayers," he said. "Maureen and I have stopped relating to each other as husband and wife." We talked about the possibility that he might be looking for another Cinderella, but he said, "Some wives discover their husband is not Prince Charming and they start looking for another Prince. It happens when they see you aren't perfect," he said. "When they see you have a wart or two."

He was telling me that he knew he wasn't perfect, but he wasn't sure of the imperfection that was causing their difficulty. Weeks later Ivan, Maureen, Joan and I were spending an evening talking things over, and I thought I saw Ivan's wart while we were discussing married life. Maureen had just said, "I get so tired of coming home after work and finding the house hasn't been cared for and my son is still in bed. Nobody seems to care about responsibility except me. One time our oldest son even threatened me and Ivan didn't do anything about it." Joan asked, "Why didn't you, Ivan?" "Because I wasn't around when it happened," he said.

Often times the I-wasn't-around-when-it-happened statement reveals a lack of love. Love is expressed in so many ways, but one way love is shown is in taking responsibility. I saw this stumbling block in Ivan and Maureen's relationship because I had been guilty of irresponsibility myself. Joan had assumed the job of paying household bills. Then, over the years, of filing the income tax return, even doing minor repairs around the house. I was caught up in heavy traveling schedules as part of my career, and it became too easy to let a competent wife take care of everything. Sometimes it's good for a wife to take care of the family finances, but in our case this went further than it should, because I was dropping everything and letting Joan pick it up. When it looked like our roof was leaking I didn't even check on that immediately, and then I realized our division of household responsibilities hadn't been a division at all. It was a subtraction of me from the real responsibility of the household.

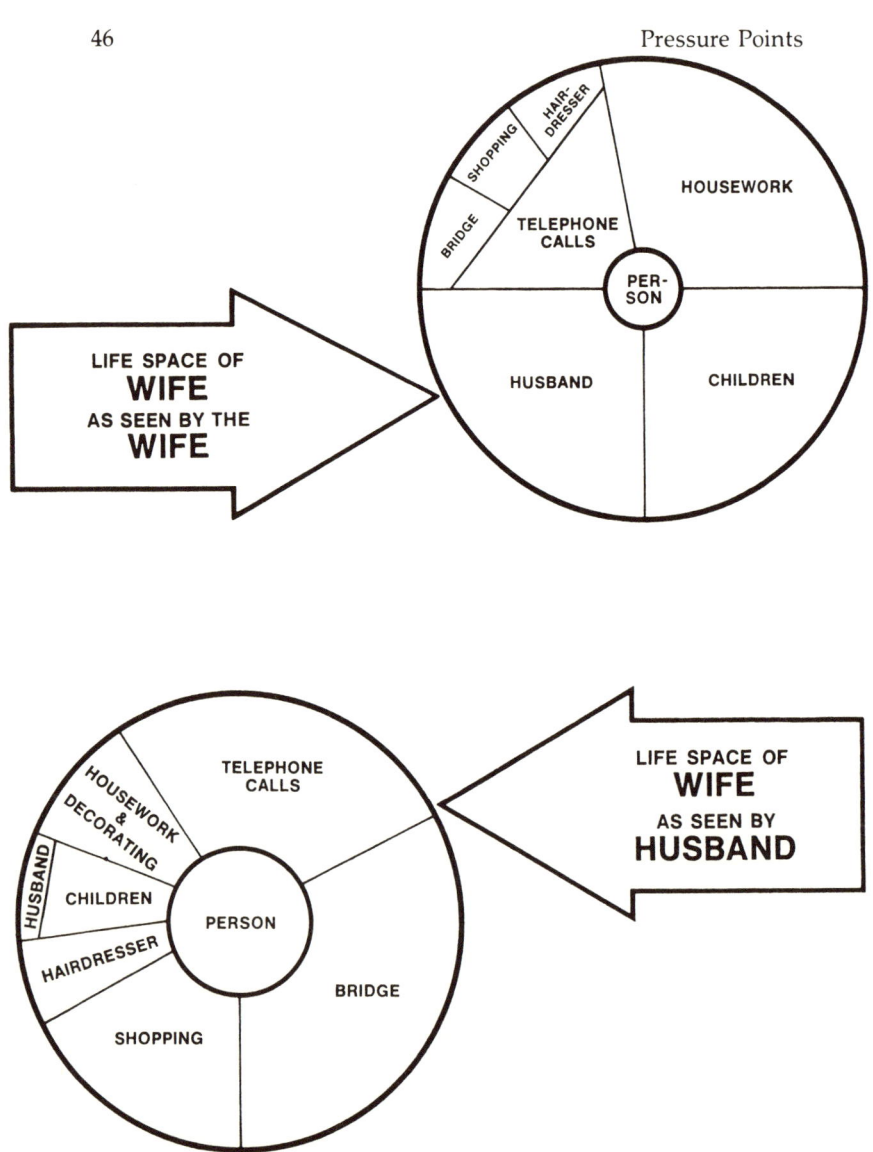

April, 1972. Dr. Margaret Gorman.
Reprinted with permission

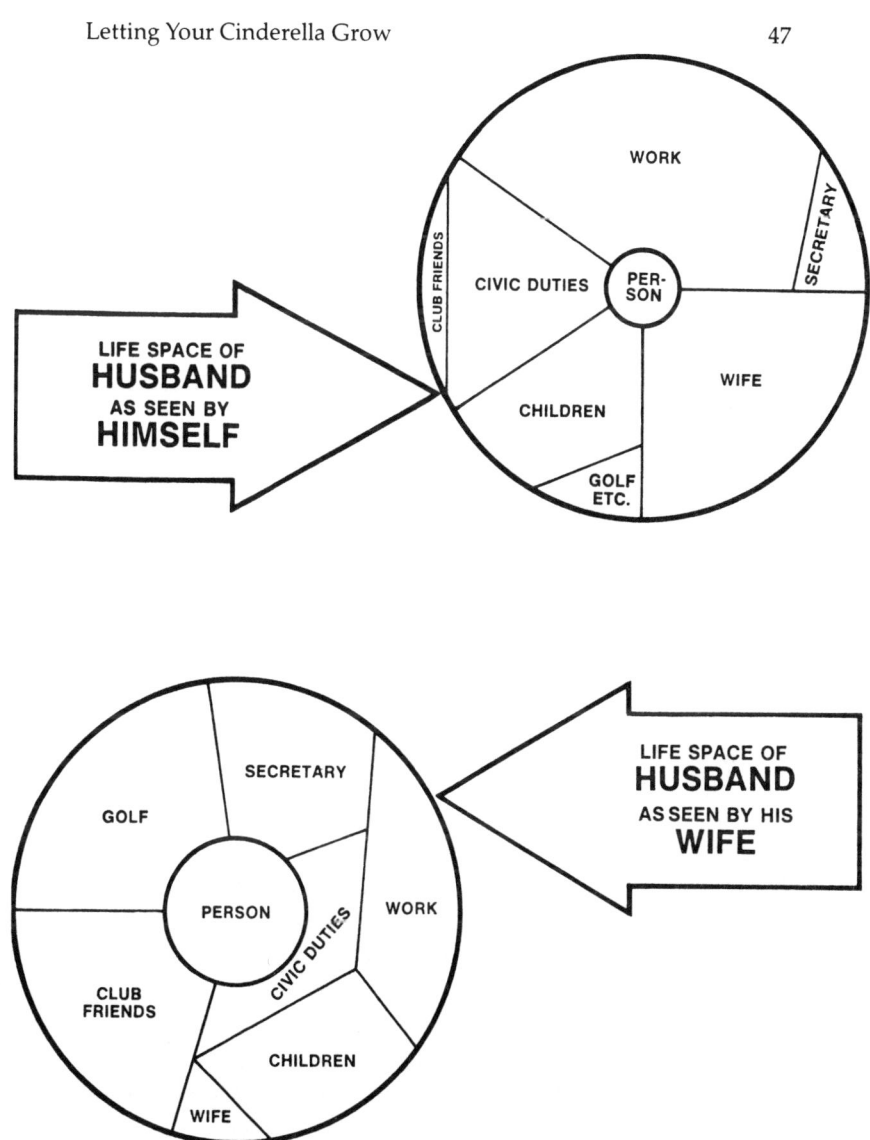

April, 1972. Dr. Margaret Gorman.
Reprinted with permission

Responsible love is shown day-to-day when a husband or wife shows he or she cares by their actions. But in Ivan and Maureen's relationship—as in ours—responsibility was lacking. There's a drawback about a lack of responsibility shown by one member of a marriage: It gives birth to irresponsibility in the other partner. Irresponsibility grows by creeping first, then crawling, and suddenly irresponsibility is the opposite of caring love. With every day of irresponsible living, we communicate in a score of ways how little we care.

And in Ivan and Maureen's case, they had finally stopped communicating. There was no longer a Cinderella and Prince Charming relationship. The relationship had reached the stage of one person asking, "Why isn't there anything physical between us anymore?" And the other asking, "Why doesn't anybody care?" The questions sound similar, but they come from a totally different world of need. I remembered the words of the discussion leader in my retreat when she said, "You don't love your wife." I was able to see how a person can look at a married couple and say, "The reason for the stress in your relationship is you aren't loving each other anymore, not on the level of *caring love*, or sacrificial love." Sometimes love can be shown only by giving up *our* wants and becoming responsible. Being responsible helps our marriage partner to become response-able. Maureen didn't want to be Cinderella anymore.

When the Ivans of the world face the *reason* their Cinderellas don't want to play that role any more, and step into the world of responsible love, we won't have as many stressful marriages. Divorces will be reduced when husbands care for their wives as they care for themselves. But this responsibility works both ways.

A successful interior designer stepped aboard a hotel limousine in Montreal with a troubled look on her face. There were just the two of us passengers so we started talking. She was heading downtown to attend a weekend conference on how to get yourself together. "I had to get away," she said, "because I'm about to be divorced. I don't know why it had to happen." As we talked the reason became more clear. "My business has been successful beyond my dreams," she said. "But my husband's business hasn't gone well. He's an architect and things have slowed down for him. A few weeks ago he fell in love with a French girl while on a separate vacation in Paris."

I found that she had been spending most of her life commuting to Montreal where she had contracts with several large firms. There hadn't been much time for her marriage because she had become devoted to her real love—her career. It was the old problem of priorities again. What are they really? What is important right now? These questions were not answered. They weren't even asked. But as we talked and I asked her if she really loved her husband she said, "Yes, I do. I'd like to save my marriage." I asked her to pray for the ability to give over her marriage to the Lord's direction; to ask him to teach her how to really love her husband. In her prayer that afternoon she asked for forgiveness and committed not only her marriage but her life to Christ's direction. As her face began to show the beginning of a new heart attitude she said, "I'm catching the next plane for New York and my husband. I'm going to show him I love him." There was no further searching for mind control or getting herself together. She had tasted a little of God's prescription for healing of relationships: Confession, forgiveness and turning away from self-love.

This design of responsible love has been mapped out for us in the New Testament. When we realize we have forgotten what responsible love is, we can confess the sin of irresponsibility. We can be forgiven and turn our direction toward the selfless love that Christ showed by his example. That kind of caring love helps stressful marriages.

Sometimes God speaks to us in unlikely places about our relationships, like hotel limousines or even a theater. Joan and I were watching a movie at Radio City Music Hall with two of our sons. The movie was about Cinderella. It was such a beautiful but unrealistic movie that God somehow used it to say to me, "You are looking at your own marriage. You've got to let your Cinderella grow. It's the way *you* can grow. You've got to learn to stop loving yourself because that's what you've been doing by holding on to a Cinderella relationship." For a while I didn't really want to let go because I wanted the adoration of my Cinderella. But I knew then that self-love isn't caring love. Self-love isn't love at all. It's a form of idolatry.

Idolatry is putting self on a pedestal. When we set someone else on a pedestal, it's because we want to be set up on one, too. An idolatrous relationship is two or more people who are really not living in commitment to each other but just living together for approval of self. Idolatry isn't love. Idolatry won't ever sacrifice self. All it will do is manipulate someone else to get its own way. This mutual self-worship is the underlying sin that erodes a marriage.

If marriage is something *we* fashion without God, it becomes self-gratification, the opposite of holy matrimony. Self-gratification, practiced long enough, is mistaken for love. Self-gratification becomes self-worship, and worship of the wrong thing has always troubled men and women. God had some strong feelings about that when he said to the children of Israel wandering in the wilderness, "I don't want you to set up any idols before me." (Today he points at our job or our marriage or us as individuals.)

Idolatry is one of the most hidden sins. It's not good for us, because it's a stressful way of life and it keeps us from a mature relationship with people and with God. Letting go of it allows us to get a better view of one more pathway to freedom from stressful living. When I said, "I'm letting Cinderella go, Lord," I began to find a new level of peace, and Joan and I began to enter into a deeper walk with each other.

A week or so later I said to Joan, "I suppose you want me to call you Joan instead of Joanie." She said, "Why don't you try?" And I said, "I love you . . . Joan."

Is your love relationship ebbing away? Are you considering dropping your partner over the side without a splash, because the relationship doesn't seem to be working for you? Consider the stress of lost relationships—and the fact that love often returns when commitment is remembered. Without commitment there is no love.

Four

Getting Together
as Parents

One of the prime causes of parental stress is not getting together over our children. But the children suffer, too, when parents disagree on the way to bring them up. The result is family turmoil. It doesn't need to be that way, because there are a number of ways to get together.

Hal and Judy Merwald work in the New York area with Young Life, a ministry to high school students, and they have found a way to be one where their family is concerned. They go away alone on their own private retreat once a year and talk about their goals as individuals, as a married couple and as parents. "We review where we've been in the last year, what each of us wants to do this year and the effect this has on our family life," Hal said to me one day. "We talk about our jobs and the way that affects all of us." Hal and Judy believe in parental unity. Living close to young people in their ministry with Young Life makes it all the more important that their own children are properly cared for. They are trying to apply the biblical principle that St. Paul wrote in Chapter 3 of his first letter to his spiritual son, Timothy. "For if a man knows not how to manage his own family, how can he take care of the church of God?" (TEV).

But there is a further question that plagues parents.

How shall we rule our own household? Sooner or later that question arises.

Listen to Bob Shealor, a Wall Street bond broker, who said one day at a men's breakfast, "Children make you think about church. For some reason I felt my children should go to church, but I felt I didn't need it. Then, after awhile, I began to feel guilty. In the high adrenaline business I'm in you run hard from 6:30 A.M. to 7:00 at night, and one day you realize your real allegiance is to your business."

"Right now," he said, "my allegiance to my family has to take precedence over allegiance even to my church. But not to God. Being sure I am a Christian father is first, and my wife is making me realize that."

This recognition of the need for parental responsiblity starts even before the birth of children. Take a look at investment counselor Jim Gardner and his wife Pauline. In their early years of marriage Jim and Pauline were preparing to have their first child. He called one morning and his voice showed his concern. "I'd like to have lunch with you," he said. "I think you can help me. It's about our forthcoming addition to the family and our relationship to church." It was several days before we got together for lunch. That gave me time to reflect on the impact of children on married people from the moment they know their own child will be born.

Having an addition to the family always has been both a blessing and a stressful time. But the stress is perhaps a little different now than it used to be. Birth isn't as ordinary an occasion as it once was, with nearly one out of two marriages breaking up. And the marriages that remain intact aren't producing as many children. At a rate of 1.8

children per marriage in the 1970's compared to 3.7 per marriage in the 1950's, children are literally going out of style! One reason is the disquieting doubt about permanence of marriage. And that's a special concern to couples thinking about having children. "We'd like to wait awhile," is the often spoken decision of young married couples—an indication of the tentative times couples are going through.

Jim Gardner had no worry about his marriage when we got together for lunch. Jim said, "We've been thinking about the christening. We don't want it to be just a family affair with a big party and pictures and gifts. We want it to be something real, but we aren't quite sure what."

I looked at Jim. He wore a well-manicured beard and well-groomed clothes, but I saw that he was troubled inside, in the same way we all are when we want to do something right but we're not sure how to go about it. "How old are you, Jim?" I asked, not knowing why. I had prayed for wisdom in talking with Jim about his forthcoming child, but I had not received a clear cut message, and it had been 11 years since the birth of our last son. "I'm 35," he said. "And my wife is 26." He smiled and said, "We have a little fun over our own generation gap. It comes up when we listen to music. She can't remember my songs." Then he hesitated for a moment. "We both are impressed with your church and we'd like to know about joining." He looked at me tentatively. "I may look prosperous, but I'm not quite there yet. I don't know about the financial commitment in membership or the requirements for christening our child there."

"All you need in order to join and to have your child

christened, as members, is to confess your need of Christ, and invite him into your life. There isn't anything else you need." I looked again at Jim as I said this and he looked a little troubled. "Have you done that, Jim?" I asked.

"No, I haven't reached there yet."

We seemed to be a long way from talking about his forthcoming child, but I went on because Jim was waiting to hear more and was listening intently.

"It's the relationship with God that's important," I said. "You can spend the rest of your life trying to figure it out and miss it completely, or you can spend the next 15 minutes and discover it. It doesn't need to be longer than that because God has no reason to delay the relationship. All you need to do is confess *you* and get yourself out of the way and let him take over." I no longer wondered why we were talking about Jim. He was experiencing what Bob Shealor had voiced and new parents know, "children make you think about God." When you really think about children you begin to think of basic relationships. Maybe that's why there was a quiet eagerness in Jim's manner. "To be a father or mother," I said, "we need to learn to be a son or daughter. All we need to do is ask ourself whether we want that kind of a relationship."

Jim quietly looked me in the eye and said, "I do."

Within a few minutes Jim had prayed as we strolled through the parking lot. There were no bells, nor whistles. I had said there might not even be a feeling, but that there would be faith. There is really no way to explain what happens to a person when he makes that commitment, because Christ touches each of us according to who we are. But he always comes in when we are real about our invitation, and that happened to Jim. What Jim Gardner instinctively seemed to know was that parents need to get together *inside*.

But a different cause of stress comes into play when one parent is deeply religious and the other is outwardly hostile, or quietly apathetic, or even interested but not yet committed. "What will we do about baptism?" is a big question for many couples who aren't together in their Christian faith. Even if there is agreement on these matters, there is the responsibility of another life to think about. Some of the questions that tug at our minds are: "What sort of life are we bringing this new creature into?" "Will we be able to afford the things our child ought to have?" "What about our freedom to just be the two of us?" These are some of the questions potential parents ask in the process of getting together. And there are some principles that can provide answers in the beginning years to make parental stress a little lighter. The first is: Learn to accept each child as a unique creation and to relate with each one as an individual. Joan and I learned this from our four sons.

We have four sons because we wanted to have a girl. That's how we got into family life without even thinking much about it. Valerie's name had been picked out for years, but never used. Kevin came along first, and as I looked at him through the hospital window I accepted what I knew I could do nothing about. We set about discovering who this new creature was, and after a few years we found out that Kevin was an artistic football player. He liked roughing and tumbling, but he also liked painting and creating, too. We didn't think there were children like that, but there he was.

When Jeff came along, I looked at him through the

hospital window and convinced myself in my prayer of acceptance that it was good to have another son, "because he'll be like Kevin and I'll understand him." But he wasn't. Jeff developed into the scholarly type over the years and was as different from Kevin in other ways as he could be. Jeff was interested in such things as science and money. These two things don't sound like interests that occur in the same boy, but they did. When Jeff reached 10 he began to ask probing questions like, "How much money do you make, dad?" That must have been a profound question because it took me three months to answer. Then I realized the reason. I didn't want Sid, my neighbor, to know how little I was making and I thought Jeff would tell.

When I finally told Jeff how much I was making, he said, "That's just about what I thought you made, dad." And that brings up the second principle about parenthood and togetherness.

Sooner or later children know our real feelings about them. We can learn the adjustments to make as parents by watching our children. They know more about us than we think, and their reactions to us often reveal where we are going wrong.

When Jeff was just a few years old, I would come home from work, swing the door open, and for some reason Jeff would immediately frown at me. After a while it dawned on me that there was something wrong in our relationship. Joan and I talked about it, and figured out that I had been reading bedtime stories to Kevin while sitting on his bed, and Jeff had to listen and watch from behind the bars of his crib. I guess to Jeff I was the father of only Kevin, and he was just an onlooker. When I realized what was happening, I said to Jeff the next night, "I'm going to read to *you* tonight, Jeff, in your crib. Because I want you to know you're my son, too." I climbed over the side, the crib creaking and groaning. Jeff, listening worriedly, mumbled something from the corner that sounded like he was ready for the worst. But somehow I got down in there all crumpled up but without breaking the crib, and finally Jeff snuggled down while I read to him. It took only one time to show Jeff I cared. Maybe because he didn't want a smashed crib.

The point is parents often don't really accept their children. Or they don't want them so soon, or so many, or they want different kinds. That's where the parental stress of not being together can start, and that kind of parental stress breeds childhood stress if it's not dealt with. Often non-acceptance of children is buried so quickly by our learned values that we accept our children in our heads and don't get around to accepting them in our hearts for years. As parents we need to get our heart together with our head if we are to avoid stressful parenthood.

There is another way in which parents need to get together. We must agree as parents that *we are in charge*. Whenever parents don't accept the responsibility of being in charge, their children suffer. Or if one parent doesn't accept the responsibility and lets the other one be the only one who corrects, there will be strained relationship between the parents—and between the children and the parents. In time, the children actually learn to hate parents who don't take charge.

You've seen a very young boy or girl who started bossing around the parents at age six, or so. Nobody is really comfortable with that, least of all the six-year-old. And

what starts out as merely an uncomfortable situation ends
up with rebellion that can go on for years. When things
aren't going right in our relationships with children, one
question to ask ourselves is, "Who's in charge here?" But
it's better to ask it quietly, honestly, before asking it aloud.
If the true answer is, "I don't know," there is likely an
undercurrent of stress going on and we may need to
repent of our unwillingness to accept the responsibility of
being a parent. Every family needs someone in charge.

It's like the story told by Jim Hayes of the American
Management Association about the father who decided to
take his family for a Sunday afternoon ride. He got everyone in the car and asked his wife, "Where do you want to
go?" "Oh, I don't care," she said. So he backed the car out
of the garage, thinking she really didn't care, and started
down the long driveway. His wife thought to herself, "He
knows I like to ride along the beach. That's probably
where we're going." His son said to himself, "Dad told me
we would go by the ice cream store next time we go for a
ride. I'll bet that's where we are going." His daughter said
to herself, "Dad promised me we would go by the zoo
Sunday afternoon." Everyone in the car already had
formed his own idea of where they were going while the
car was still going down the driveway. When the father
turned right at the end of the drive, his wife said, "What
did you do that for?" That's when the trouble started,
because there really hadn't been agreement.

The place to get agreement on a Sunday drive is in the
garage, especially if you have a long driveway. The length
of the driveway determines the degree of mental set. As
parents, the longer we *think* there is togetherness when
there isn't, the harder it is to accept another direction, and

the harder it is for the children. There is less stress in family life when the parents are together, not only in the beginning, concerning how many children there will be, but later concerning the direction of the children.

But something different happens after 10 years or so in many marriages. In the earlier years, the husband often leads the way in family matters, but sometimes the wife takes a stronger role regarding the children in the later years. If a wife sees her husband relinquishing his direction she may interpret it as a lack of interest and become resentful that he isn't providing the fatherly support needed in directing their growing family. It works the same the other way around. A wife who gives approval for something when she knows her husband is against it, contributes to a spirit of rebellion in the family. And rebellion is contagious. It can start with anyone. In my case, I rebelled even at the use of the word rebellion by Joan when she corrected the children. I felt she was taking over.

The problem of authority is a difficult one where husband and wife are concerned. Too often a husband wants to accept St. Paul's advice concerning the man being the head of the woman and overlooks the admonition that this is to be worked out in a life of mutual submission, "in honor preferring one another." The words, "because I said so," seldom work with a wife or husband, because it's a sure sign that togetherness is gone. A contest of wills is not a marriage. Neither is it a sign of love. In parent-child relationships, love works on the foundation of authority. With husbands and wives, the scriptural authority of a husband is based upon his sonship to God. Christ is the model for this, and he mixed authority with love.

When our third son came along, I learned a valuable lesson about authority and love. Drew wasn't the scholarly type at first. In his early years he was the kind of boy who would drag the neighbors' used Christmas trees into our backyard to sell. He was creative, but he had one or two things to learn about marketing. I did the thing most fathers do. I said in a thundering voice, "Drew, get into the backyard and take those trees back." But Drew went into a frozen state, and he certainly didn't go out and clear the yard. I guess I yelled too loudly and froze his ability to respond. Then I picked another approach. I put my hand on his shoulder and stood beside him, looking at the backyard. "Drew," I said earnestly, but quietly, "the back yard's a mess. If you clean it up . . ." I paused to see if we were together. "You won't get a spanking." A look of understanding spread over Drew's face and he went right into the back yard and cleaned it up. I discovered that a basic need of children is filled when parents realize their children aren't the enemy. The back yard is the enemy. When we keep that in mind, throughout our lives, we can stand with our arm around our son or daughter, and point out what needs to be done. It can work with husbands and wives, too. When authority stands alongside rather than in front, a togetherness relationship can happen *without throwing authority away.*

There are special times to develop responsible relationships like this. We discover them when we learn to look for life's fruitful moments. Our last son, Trevor, in his early years, was the most articulate son of our four boys, but that probably was due to the fact that he was the smallest and had to use the power of words with his bigger brothers. Or maybe it was because by age seven he had

had 17,000 hours of television education. One Saturday, concerned about his lack of playtime, somehow we unplugged him from the television set to go swimming. He stood at the edge of the pool strapping on a life vest, probably the first time he had ever tried to put one on.

As he was about to jump into the deep part of the pool, I stood, waiting on the walk nearby. No doubt the life jacket would have protected him, but I wanted to share in the experience that was about to happen. He jumped in with all the abandon of a little guy who doesn't know what fear is, and slipped down deep in the water. As he broke through the surface again I was standing at the edge of the pool, looking him straight in the eye, and he yelled. "Emergency! Emergency!" (We used to say "help" when I was a kid.)

Instead of jumping in, I showed him how to depend on the life jacket. That was a fruitful moment in our relationship because we both received something from it. I particularly learned a profound principle of relationship: Although we get busy with one thing or another that needs to be done, if we sense that a meaningful moment is about to happen, we must stop everything we are doing and wait for that moment to occur. We need to *be there* with all of ourselves, and learn what it really means to get beside someone when they need help. That isn't possible all the time because we are too busy. But when we *are* around, we can learn to shut out the unimportant things.

Even in the middle of stress, fruitful moments for parents are close at hand—when there is a difference of opinion about the way a son or daughter should be cared for; when our wife or husband feels we aren't carrying the load, or feels that we aren't aware that a son or daughter's actions are a cry for help. As a husband or wife, we capture fruitful moments when we are willing to share concerns with our mate.

One day Joan and I were out for a drive. I had not seen the anguish she was carrying inside for one of our sons because I hadn't seen the danger he was in. Instead, I had been struggling to maintain my viewpoint and there was a deep gulf between us over how to handle him. As the car broke over the top of a hill, I suddenly realized that I must stop fighting and confess that I didn't have all the answers. That was the beginning of our getting together again in our handling of a troubled son.

Later that day we found out that someone had felt a strong urge to stop what she was doing to pray for Joan and me. She didn't know why, or what to pray for, but she prayed for us anyway, at just the time we were out for our drive. Fruitful moments happen too, when we stop what we are doing and respond to what God wants us to do. They occur to anyone—even to someone who doesn't know the problem, but is willing to stop and pray when another person is brought to mind.

But stress that comes from unresolved relationships is relieved when we get together with each other, *especially* when we disagree, and say, "I'm right here beside you, and I'm trying to understand." If we don't know what to say or how to work out the problem, we need to remember that the Source of Wisdom in all our relationships is available in *the middle* of our disagreements. All we need to say is "emergency," and open our eyes. Then we see that God has been standing by, looking deep into our lives and saying, "I've been here all the time. If you will listen, I'll tell you how to get out of this. I'll show you how to get together."

But we must remember that God speaks powerfully and he speaks in many ways—sometimes in a still, small voice; sometimes through a person's prayer (even when they aren't around); and sometimes through someone who is standing right beside us. Our responsibility is to make certain we are listening. When we do that we have a better opportunity to live together in harmony. According to Phillip's translation of the second chapter of Philippians, we are to live as though we have one mind and one spirit between us. We are never to act from motives of rivalry, or personal vanity, ". . . but in humility think more of each other than you do of yourselves." How do we do that? By dropping what interests only us as an individual. By stopping what we are doing for our sake and entering into someone else's deep water for their sake. But we must remember that we aren't the life jacket. That's where true humility comes in. *Our job is to remember that we can't lick family stress alone.*

When our sons and daughters enter the middle teen years we discover there is a special need for spiritual answers to stressful living. We will look at these stressful years next.

Five

Surviving the Middle-Teen Itch

As a parent, going through your son's or daughter's middle-teen years is like riding in a car that is shifting into passing gear on a dirt road. But it starts with your son or daughter's foot on the gas pedal, not yours. You hear the roar of the engine, feel a burst of energy, see a cloud of dust, and everybody in the car worries until you all arrive at your destination safely.

The sudden shift of a middle-teen takes many families by surprise, but it has been going on for centuries. The shift is really the result of a teen-age itch that develops over several months, and virtually everyone feels it. And we can't ignore an itch. We must do something about it, and it's how we react to it that raises our tension—or helps us survive. There is little doubt about middle-teen difficulty occurring, so we might as well get ready if we can.

Using the analogy of shifting into the passing gear, here's a more complete picture of what happens. Our teenage son or daughter stomps on the gas pedal while we reach for the brake and grip the wheel tighter. Tension takes over as we bring the car to a sliding stop, and nobody looks out the window to see where we are. In family life, everything seems to have suddenly gone wrong, much like the incident I have described. But it doesn't need to go wrong.

Call the middle-teen shift what we like—teen-age rebellion, identity crisis, or just growing pains—it's important to call time out for a while when it happens, and ask, "What's going on here?" Tension can be reduced when a family realizes that the itch and the shift are part of growing up. At age 15, something is going to happen, because it's *supposed* to happen. It usually lasts no more than a year, maybe two, and if things work out right, the teenager doesn't go back in the same gear. He or she shifts into early adulthood (not mature adult-hood, just early adulthood), and the parents learn that it's different to be a father or mother of an early adult. Much of the stress is in working out this new relationship. Some teen-agers and parents shift with a jolt, some with relative ease. Some delay the shift for five or 10 years. Some children, and parents, never grow up. Part of the reason is that, like most itches, we don't know exactly when the middle-teen experience is going to come. Even though it often occurs around 15, it could come a little earlier or later, and the expression is somewhat different with each son or daughter in the same family.

When our oldest son, Kevin, ran away at 15, Joan and I were as lost as he was. We didn't know which way to turn. When we remembered that wisdom comes to those who seek it, as explained in the first chapter of James, we got through one of the most stressful times of our family life. Jeff, our second son, went through the middle-teen itch a year or so later. We never knew until he was 19 that he, too, wanted to run away, just a year or two after Kevin did. Circumstances changed that, however, because we moved from Long Island to Kansas City. In a sense we all ran away, and began to get a little closer as a family. It wasn't until years later that we realized Jeff's change had occurred. That was in his junior year in high school. From our point of view he had been bored to the point of apathy. We hadn't known whether he would toss out all his good marks in school, drift away from the years of responsible schoolwork and miss out on his college dreams altogether. Besides that, he had decided showers were a waste of time and energy. We had been in a slough of despondency for a while, but Jeff pulled out of it. Then Drew went into it, yet in a different way. Drew ran away, but his body was still around. We didn't know he had run away. There are a lot of teen-agers who have run away while staying at home. Most don't really want to run away. They want attention. Here's how we discovered that to be true with Drew.

When Joan found a small leather box in Drew's top dresser drawer and saw that it was equipment for smoking marijuana or hash, she brought it to me. "Don," she said with anxiety in her voice, "what do you think about this?" I looked and knew Drew and I had to talk. When he came to my room I showed him the box and asked, "Do you want to tell me about his?" "Yes," he said, "I do." I thought there was a certain relief in his voice as he continued.

"Two years ago I stopped smoking marijuana, dad. A neighbor kid supplied it. I had been smoking it for about nine months. Then I began to see what was happening to me, and to my friends, so I stopped. Some of them went on to heavier stuff, but I haven't been going around with them for two years now."

When he named the others I realized that I hadn't seen them for a long time, so I felt Drew was telling the truth. Over the next several days I checked with the school authorities and the police and found that everything fit the way Drew had said. My reason for checking was to stop dope traffic that had grown all around us so that Trevor, our 10-year-old, wouldn't get involved. While doing that I developed a new respect for Drew and I thanked God for giving him the wisdom to stop.

A few days after our conversation, Drew took a 15-cent item from the school cafeteria and was caught. When I appeared in the assistant principal's office he said, "Your son seems to be asking for attention." Drew was now 15. He had run away, inside, a few months ago and now he wanted someone to notice.

Now that we were facing the problem of our third teenager, Joan and I went to talk with our pastor, our neighbors, and our other sons who had gone through it earlier. Kevin had some helpful thoughts. He was now 20 and married, already a homeowner with a minimum amount of financial help from Joan and me. "Don't let up on strictness, Dad," he said, "but don't try to make him into another you. That won't work." I had come to appreciate Kevin in a new way as I dropped in to see him in Cheyenne, Wyoming from time to time and began to talk to him as adult to adult. His Air Force experience there had not been easy for him but it had been good.

Later, Joan and I talked with Jeff, now a well-groomed sophomore, home from college during the Christmas vacation. After two years of physics and math at Houghton, a small liberal arts Christian college, Jeff had begun to really develop awareness, socially as well as intellectually.

"I think part of the answer is in doing things with each son before he reaches 13, dad. Togetherness trips like we've had—camping and the trip to California were good. But each son has a special interest that is him and he needs you to enter into that world with him. Don't let parenthood stop at telling Drew what tasks must be done. Don't let it be just delegating things and then going away. I think knowing your son at 12 is important." Jeff stopped then and reflected, "I don't know about girls. . . ."

I asked my neighbor Art about girls. "They're always primping in the bathroom, Don," he said, "and they're a real worry when they come out. So many things can go wrong, on a date, for instance. I worry a lot." Then he got serious. "I think it's important for a mother to be especially close to daughters and a father to be especially close to sons."

Our pastor made yet another point. "Don't try to be a buddy. Don't try to please your children all the time. They will grow up to hate you if you do that. Be a father. Stand against their desire for too much freedom, too soon. They need restrictions and actually want them. Give them the security of standing fast. Let them know you are praying for them and that you believe in tough love—because you know more about life than they do."

I thought about the good advice I had received. Then I began to reflect on the fact that the difficult teen-age years seem to occur both in intensely religious and nonreligious families as well. It doesn't seem to matter what the background or denomination or faith. In discussions with a Presbyterian minister I found these reflections on his early years: "I was a real rebel. At different times I drove a motorcycle west, took my father's car out of state and caused a lot of trouble in my family before I got out of the teen-age rebellion. And I grew up in a fundamental Baptist environment."

Joan's parents were nominal Episcopalians. She didn't leave the state or join a motorcycle gang, but she rebelled in a more passive way. "I just felt my folks didn't understand me," she said. "I felt I was a lot smarter than they were. They had paid for my voice lessons, piano lessons, tap-dancing and ballet, and I guess I thought I was outgrowing them. I used to go into my room and play the piano all by myself."

The teen-age experiences we have been reviewing are all individual, as are the bits and pieces of good advice. The parents of a middle-teen can get all the advice needed. The problem soon becomes an introspective thing. "How much of this is my fault?" we ask, or we throw up our hands as the parents did in the Broadway production of *Fiddler on the Roof,* when they compared rearing children to growing flowers. Planting flowers is so much easier than having children. When you plant a buttercup or a pansy, it grows up a buttercup or a pansy. The question is, "Now that I know so much, which way do I turn?"

To answer that, it may help to review one or two of the big lies that parents have believed. A big lie is a lie that sounds so much like truth that you base your behavior on it. Here's one big lie that has caused a family to stumble during the middle-teen itch: "All a father needs to do is take care of his wife. By making her happy, she will see that the children are happy." I believed this lie for years, partly because it was pronounced by a nationally renowned clinical psychologist in lectures given around the United States. There is a shade of truth in this notion, but it absolves the husband of his fatherhood responsibilities. It's similar to the saying, "The best thing a father can do for his children is love their mother." That has a nice ring to it, but it doesn't help the teen-age itch. Nor does it help you when you turn it around: "The best thing a mother can do for her children is love their father," or "All a mother needs to do is take care of her husband . . . he will see that the children are happy." The thinness of these notions becomes more apparent when you change the perspective.

Here's another big lie: "Let the teen-agers decide things on their own. They'll learn by doing things wrong." That's a true statement, but people don't usually learn how to do things right by doing things wrong. They learn how to do things wrong.

There are other big lies that we've all believed and tried. And there are words of good advice, too. There just isn't a neat little checklist of things to do that produces the right answer every time. But there is a basic approach that works, and lets us find a workable solution in the middle of the problem. It's the second great commandment of Jesus, "You should love your neighbor as you love yourself." Joan repeated that to me one night at the kitchen table, but she said it in *our* context as we were trying to determine how to handle one of our sons in the middle of his rebellion. I had been trying to figure it out all by myself in a state of personal rebellion—the covert kind that says, "I can handle this one, Lord." Joan said, "It's not any one thing you can do, Don. It's your heart attitude that needs changing. You need to love your family as you do yourself." Those were words of truth for me and I knew it. I prayed then as I had not prayed before and I went to Drew and told him I was trying to learn how to love him as I loved me. Something began to happen then. Drew's difficult time didn't immediately go away but it got less difficult that night, and in time Drew became a very responsible, hard working and loving teen-age son.

Loving a son or daughter in the midst of his or her rebellion gives us a better understanding of God's love for us when we rebel. The first step for a parent who has a rebellious son or daughter is to look within and ask for discernment of any personal rebellion. When you sincerely ask for it you get it. I then began to apply Christ's teaching to one of my closest neighbors—my rebellious son. It works with sons or daughters of any age. It worked with Trevor at 10 when he had been fighting school authority. He was trying to con the teachers and he could charm them out of their socks for the moment, but he was losing the war. When I sat beside a troubled 10-year-old, and asked God to forgive him for his heart attitude—but to forgive me too, for mine—he healed us both. And that was a new beginning—before the middle-teen itch had a chance to develop.

Six

Watch Out for Controlling People

We've all met controlling people in our lives. They come in all sizes and shapes. Some of them are occasional acquaintances and some are in our own families. Few of them add real value. All of them add stress to our lives.

A controlling person is someone who uses another person for personal gain. We've all been controlling in our actions at times; when we've tried to raise funds for a charity or found help for a neighborhood club or conducted a touchy business meeting. That's acceptable behavior to most of us. It's even desirable, if we feel the cause is right. But *controlling people* are never desirable, because they rob us of ourselves. In the long run they fail to do good for others even though it may seem at times that they are trying to do good.

Let's look at some controlling behavior. The first example of control is a father who wanted his son to go to college even though his son had no desire to go. They talked things over for weeks until the son finally said flatly, "I'm not going, dad." Then the father finally gave up, realizing he had wanted his son to go to college mainly because he had not graduated himself. For a while, the father had been a controlling person. Whether or not it would have been good for the son to go to college was not the real issue; the father's motive was more self-interest than concern for his son's future. A major cause of stress among college age people is controlling parents who won't listen to their sons or daughters. College people need to learn how to live their own lives, not to be their parents' alter ego.

Another controlling person is Theresa, who won't let her daughter and son-in-law raise their own children. From the beginning, Theresa had an idea of the way her grandchildren should be raised, and she made it clear what should happen right from the start. Finally, Theresa's son-in-law put his foot down. He'd had enough of someone else raising his children and banned Theresa from the premises. It was stressful before the ban and it was stressful after, because of the loss of relationship. If Theresa could learn to love her children and grandchildren for *their* sake it would reduce the frustration for everyone.

Here is another example: a father who expresses his control by wanting to obligate his daughter. By rushing to loan her money at the drop of a hat and showering her with gifts, he attempts to keep her his little girl. This, Papa's-going-to-make-life-all-right approach will likely either stunt his daughter's growth or make her despise him in the end, or both.

Another example of a controlling mother is one who can't accept her son's decision to get married. The idea of moving over for another woman in her son's life is unbearable, so she finds a way to harpoon every girl that comes along. Or take a look at a mother who has never approved of the husband her daughter picked. "He'll never be good enough for my daughter," she thinks to herself, but the attitude alone lets him know her feelings in a score of unspoken ways.

These are just a few examples of controlling people. There are others, including parents who won't let their children grow up, or people who spend the greater share of their marriage trying to change their mate. There are still other controlling people who "freeze" or hold their mates in an old mistake, because they really don't want to forgive. Some controlling people don't want others to change toward them, because they want to feel persecuted or hurt or superior. By freezing a relationship they can hold on to a self-image of being the wronged one. But this causes internal strife for everyone and ends up in a family civil war. These civil wars cost a great deal. They are stressful rather than productive, because people don't like to be changed or held in an old position by others. Civil wars are unproductive not only because of the loss of time and energy, but also a loss of freedom to really enjoy each other.

But hard-core controlling people don't stop at family conquests. Have you ever worked for a boss whose manifest objective seemed to be to make you into an image of himself? There are papa bosses and mama bosses who gather industrial sons and daughters around them or send them out on key assignments to extend their own influence. That works today just as it has for hundreds of years. But it works today only because there are people who allow it. The sin of controlled relationships on or off the job is not one-sided; it is mutual, because the one who is controlled allows it to happen.

Here is what happened in one instance of boss control.

For more than a year an educator kept saying to a subordinate teacher, "You've got to teach your classes the way I do." The teacher had been teaching for years and was effective in the classroom, but the boss was bound to change her approach in order to dominate the relationship. Finally, after several earnest but unproductive talks, she wrote a letter to her boss and said, "I owe you the dedication to meet our teaching objectives but you've got to give me the freedom to accomplish them in a different way from yours. I can't do it your way and be as effective. I'll meet the objectives and do a good job. I promise. As long as I do that you owe me the liberty of letting me do it a different way." She never sent the letter. She handed it to her boss and asked him to read it on the spot so they could talk about it. By doing that, she resisted the control but agreed to the discipline of getting the job done right.

There is a difference between discipline—or training—and control. Control is forcing your way for your sake, not for the good of the job or the person's development. Control is bad. Training and discipline are good.

The way out of the controlling person dilemma is to ask. "What's going on here? What are the objectives? How can we get our egos out of the way?"

But what about a *self-controlling* person who is trying to atone for an old sin by levying his own punishment? A middle age woman—we'll call her Janet—did something wrong in her youth. She never was caught and she carried the guilt around for years. Then, years after she was married, she started having a series of illnesses, accidents and woeful circumstances. No one could define why these things were happening to her, but the pattern was too clear to be a chance thing. Sometimes people like

Janet, who are never caught for doing something wrong, carry guilt around all their lives. Seeing no way to settle the score or make the wrong right, they develop accident proneness or run themselves down so they become illness-prone. Often they don't know what is happening, even though they are controlling the very things that cause stressful living. There is a way out of this kind of stressful living, but it isn't through self-control.

Self-control is one of the notions that is worshiped in today's world. We idolize those whom we think are most in control. The ultimate person seems to be the cool, controlled man or woman who keeps everything about self in perfect subjection. But this presumes that we know what is good for us, when in reality many of us don't. The cool, self-controlled person may have forgotten how to be warm and open and accepting of love from someone who could help, and probably doesn't realize that he may even be helped by helping others. Janet's control *is causing* her lifelong stress. And the cool, controlled person isn't learning what real relationship is. Both are "in control," and losing out.

Where does this human preoccupation with self-control come from? A certain amount comes from the way we were created by God, who knew when he created us that we would need the ability to take charge if we were to be fruitful and multiply, and care for the earth. That is also where human ego comes in. It was created by God for his purposes, as a part of us. We can't pry it apart from ourselves even if we want to. But we do err when we worship our ego instead of merely using it as he intended. That's the nemesis of humanity: using our gifts for selfish purpose. When we willfully wrest from God control of self for our gain, without regard to the kingdom that God intended, we are trying to control something that really isn't ours. It's like misappropriating funds. That's something that our human laws put us in prison for. In the kingdom of heaven, misappropriating the gifts of the kingdom is handled in the same way, except that we lock ourselves out of the kingdom and into our self-made prison. That is the real story of Genesis. Having lost our freedom then by locking ourselves out of real friendship by our own control, we extend our controlling behavior and rob someone else of their freedom, without even knowing what we are doing. And so the imprisonment process goes on.

Where did we learn control? From the original couple. From Eve, when she thought she really ought to take things into her own hands, and then wanted Adam as an accomplice. From Adam, when he agreed. The birth of "ego stress," as we know it today, occurred when the first woman and the first man lost their relationship with God and started a chain of events handed down from parents to children until today. One of the prime causes of stress—loss of relationship—was accomplished by the first couple when they traded relationship for control. This "control nature" was built into the fiber of our way of life by us. We have taught ourselves to be individuals. We always want to be in control. Unfortunately, we believe we are. But one of the most profound truths in all history is clearly stamped across the pages of life, threaded through the biblical accounts of Old Testament mankind and clarified by Christ thoughout his life. *We never are in control.* To spend our lives trying to be in ultimate control, or to control others, is to be controlled by the same serpent that manipulated Eve and promised Christ his own kingdom. If Satan can get us to do what he wants, he is in control. We are not.

But let's look more closely at our own world today. What happens in *our* relationships where control creeps in? There are many names for what happens: manipulation, overprotection, obligation and domination, to name a few. If our parents are still telling us how to run our homes, after we have established a separate life, domination may be at work. Parental domination of children who are adults is a special problem in family life. It is accomplished by obligating them, overprotecting or manipulating them. All of these approaches are not healthy if practiced long enough, because they stunt growth.

But how should we act when we are controlled? How do we get out of the stressful box someone has put us in? One way is by learning how not to be a controlling person ourselves. Or by releasing our desire to control someone else, or by asking prayerfully for the ability to let God handle our family relationships, rather than trying to change our parents, children or spouse. There are five specific steps we can take to begin the healing of stressful control in our family and work life. We can:

• Forgive each controlling person in our life (parents, spouse, boss, neighbor) remembering that Christ said the Father will not forgive us if we cannot forgive others.

• Ask for a revelation of controlling behavior in our own lives, and for forgiveness for each controlling relationship we are holding, knowing that God is faithful and just to forgive us our sins and to cleanse us from all unrighteousness.

• Invite his presence in all of our relationships and ask him to let us be an open channel of his love.

• Practice unconditional love by letting the persons we

have been controlling know we love them *without any change* on their part. This doesn't mean we condone their behavior, just that we love them as they are. It helps to remember that while we are yet sinners, God loves us— unconditionally.

• Realize that it is God's job to change people. And he doesn't do it just by force. By telling God we aren't going to try to do his work for him we are relieved of a stressful burden.

These five steps can release us and drop the chains from others at the same time. They can help us realize one of the basic teachings of Christ in the Sermon on the Mount. "Don't criticize people, and you will not be criticized. For you will be judged *by the way you criticize others*, and the measure you give will be the measure you receive" (*Matthew* 7:1; *Phillips* italics added). Controlling behavior begets controlling behavior. It is the most deadly form of criticism.

There is also something called self-righteousness. It includes thinking we know better than someone else what is good for them, and letting them know it. We cause people to miss the kingdom this way. But self-righteousness is different from the discipline we owe our children. That must happen if we are to do our part as parents. Nor does it have anything to do with saying— with love—something to a friend, in or out of church, when they are doing something wrong. There is a provision for that. The point is we can be honest without dominating. We can discipline without robbing someone of the unique creation God wants that person to become. With this awareness in mind we can go to someone in an attitude of honest love and tell them our concerns. But it is always right to ask, prayerfully, "Am I doing this for my benefit or for that person's benefit?" That helps make it clear whether we are controlling or not. Sometimes it is good to get an opinion about our real motivation from someone else not involved, before we correct another. Sometimes it is good to stay home and watch out for the controlling person we are. And freedom from the stress of being controlled ourselves comes quickest when our own controlling behavior is dropped over the side, without a splash. Then we can begin to learn to love our parents, our families and our neighbors as ourselves. We need all the help we can get in that. Fortunately, we don't have to do it alone. In fact we can't possibly do it alone. Certainly not if we have been hiding from ourselves.

Seven

Are You Hiding from Yourself?

I ran into a colleague the other day. He had just been transferred to the building where I work. We were hurrying up the stairs and I said to him, "Oh, you're here now!" "I guess so," he said, "but is anybody ever where they are?" He was poking a little fun at the old physical law of continuity that says, "Everybody has to be someplace." But when I thought about his fun-comment more seriously I realized that he was really raising one of the more stressful questions we need to face in life: "Where am I?" That question can be troublesome because most of us at some time in life are not quite sure of the answer. We are not quite sure what is going on at work, nor in our complex society. Nor are we quite sure of what is going on inside ourselves.

By now it is becoming clear, unlikely as it may seem, that we can actually experience stress without knowing it. After reading some of the stress concepts discussed in Part Ore, a woman from California wrote that they "opened my eyes to the stress I did have and not know. . ."

There are at least three ways in which this not knowing can come about. One is called "living up to our ego ideal."

Another is "giving orders to ourselves," and a third is "stifling our feelings." We'll explore all three in an attempt to overcome the costly stress of being a hidden person. Hidden people not only hide their feelings from others, they hide feelings from themselves. They spend a good portion of their lives trying to be someone else and living stressful lives in the process.

Here is how living up to our ego ideal can affect us, drawing from psychologist Dr. Harry Levinson's illustration: Suppose my wife Joan and I had invited you and your spouse or a friend to a party this Saturday night and we told you we have invited all the prominent cultural and social people in our town. Let's imagine it is now Saturday night. For some reason you have accepted our invitation and you have just parked your car quite a distance from our home, at the end of a long string of cars. Now you are walking up our long driveway. Both you and your escort are dressed in your finest as you look at our home, yet you feel just a little uncomfortable. Perhaps because our home is a palatial mansion. (It's not. It's a mansion only in this illustration, in case you really do come to see us.)

Now you are standing on our front porch. It's not really a porch, it's a sweeping veranda and you are standing between two huge white columns and you are ringing the doorbell. No one comes to the door for a long time and now you are beginning to feel even more uncomfortable.

Finally, the door swings open but it's not Joan or I. It's a butler, dressed just like the one in *Gone with the Wind,* and he says, "Come right in." You step inside the foyer and, seeing no one you know, you get a glass of something to drink from a passing waiter. You see that the real party is taking place in a large room through a big archway. Now, walking through the archway you are experiencing more feelings about yourself. You still don't see me, nor any one you know, so you pick out a couple across the room that look a little lonely and you stroll across the long expanse, thinking of all the sophisticated things you want to say. When you reach the lonely looking couple you say, "Nice weather we're having." But somehow you had planned to say something more sophisticated, and in the middle of your feelings about this you spill your drink on the rug. Instantly, you know this is a very expensive rug, and at that moment I arrive on the scene and you say rather loudly to your spouse or friend, "What did you do that for?"

This imaginary incident serves to remind us that we will do almost anything to get out of the limelight when our actions do not support our notion of how sophisticated or smooth we are. Often, we will shift the attention to someone else when we don't look good. One of the strongest motivations there is in our society is the urge to find out how good we are and to play down our unwelcome behavior. We have an ego ideal tucked away inside us and we spend a good deal of our lives trying to live up to it. This is not the strongest motivation there is, just the one that most people are possessed with. It is stressful because it frustrates us when we don't live up to our ego ideal. And the gap between our actions at a party, or anywhere else, causes us stress.

How do you feel when you have just spilled something on the floor in public? Most of us feel angry, but it's a different anger than if we spill something in the kitchen when no one is around. Then we are angry perhaps because there is extra work in cleaning it up, but in public we are more likely angry at the circumstance that shows us as a clumsy person. Or, more honestly, we are angry at ourselves for dropping our own mask of sophistication.

All of us have a mask. If I were to show up at your house on the wrong night for a party and you were to tell me at the door, "Oh no, it's tomorrow night," my inclination would be to say, "I know that. I just happened to be in the area and I thought I would stop by." This I've-got-life-all-together mask is a common one for many. Take men for instance. They don't like to admit they can't afford something, because their role is to provide. They like to have people know they are a success in a financial way. But women wear masks too, very often related to their ability to run a spotless kitchen, especially if they are not employed outside the home. More recently, women are putting on other masks as revealed in the following statement, written by a woman, that appeals to a woman's ego in today's world of the liberation movement, "Whatever women do, they must do twice as well as men. Fortunately, that's not difficult."

A good deal of our male or female stress comes from the struggle to keep our mask in place. If we are successful and we somehow succeed in almost living up to our ego ideal, or our image of ourself, we adjust our goals higher and race after a new, higher notion of how good we are. This achievement race has some good in it, because we get things done that way, but it is bad if that's all our living amounts to. After a while the achievement race gets to be a wearing one. *We know where we are going but we forget where we are.* We tend to think of ourselves only in terms of what we are becoming. Along the way we lose the ability to relate, not only to our families but to ourselves.

Along with this strong motivation of the ego ideal is the technique we have developed of giving orders to ourselves. Most orders are forgotten by us because they deal with behavior we don't want to recognize as a part of us. Our orders deal with the gap between our ego ideal and where we are right now. Generally, we give ourselves orders to protect ourselves from hurt. Here are some examples of feelings that resulted in such orders.

Fear of Losing a Loved One

A widow remarried after several years and had a child by her second marriage. She became fearful that her child might be killed and didn't want to let him out of her sight. As a result she overprotected her son and herself. Years before, when her first husband died, she had given herself an order that she would never let herself be hurt again.

Fear of Rejection

A woman had been rejected by one of her parents when she was young. When she married she held her husband away in a "safe" relationship so that she wouldn't be too hurt if he ended up rejecting her. She didn't even know that was the reason for her distant relationship with her husband until she had been married for years. Her order: Don't allow yourself to be hurt again by rejection.

Achievement

A young man who was born in a rural setting was not skilled in hard labor, athletic games or other activities of his countryside environment. He became a loner and when he entered business years later he spent his career proving to himself that he could be a succes on his own terms without depending on anyone else. It wasn't until he reached his forties that he began to realize he wasn't a well-rounded team player on the job and it began to limit his effectiveness. He had given himself an order that he would play a solitary game and become a success. Money became the way he kept score. But his lack of relational attention made him a lonely person.

Willfullness

A little girl was told sternly by her father to stop salting her food so much. She never salted her food again until her forties. She had given herself an order, but hers was a different kind. She deprived herself for years, out of spite, and to protect her own willfullness. In a way she was saying, "If I can't salt my food as much as I want, I won't salt it at all."

All of us have given ourselves an order at some time in our lives. With young boys it's often the game called, "If we don't play my way, I'll take my ball and go home." With adults it's another game. These ego sins cause us to withdraw from relationships, and the inability to be open and accepting and relaxed with ourselves dries up our lives as well as the lives of others around us.

The other area of exploration mentioned earlier is the tendency to stuff our real feelings. We have a notion that it is not Christian to get angry so we say, "I'm not really angry; I'm just annoyed." This dishonesty with ourselves occurs so fast at times that we don't even recognize the feeling passing by. Some of the expressions that go with this lightning-like ability we develop are, "It doesn't matter," "What's the difference?" or "I'll think about it tomorrow." These often are rationalizations to tell ourselves there is no reason to be angry, so we tell ourselves that we are not angry. And in that way we push down our anger, not even recognizing that it has been stored inside. But anger must come out or it will be expressed in some other way—often against someone who had nothing to do with the cause of anger in the first place.

Paul the Apostle gave some advice to the Ephesian people that applies to anyone guilty of stuffing anger inside. "Be ye angry and sin not: let not the sun go down upon your wrath: neither give place to the devil" (Ephesians 4:26 KJV). How does that apply to us? If we are angry we are to be honest about it. We are to be careful that our anger is not the sinful anger of a hurt ego, pride or bad temper, as opposed to anger at wrongdoing. And we are not to go to sleep still angry. If we sleep with our anger still within we may bury it deep down inside where it will be carried around the next day, out of mind *but in our heart.* That way we are giving a part of our life over to occupation by sin. That kind of buried anger keeps us from living life free of the overburden of ego stress.

The healing of ego stress is God's specialty. Ego stress comes from anger, fear and selfishness, among other things. It is all self and no commitment. How can we be free of it? Not by remedies that we can apply by ourselves, because usually we don't even know that we have this dis-ease called ego stress. We need someone outside ourselves who knows us and who loves us and who is willing to be painfully honest to help us. We need real friends who will covenant with us to help us be free. A true friend is someone who really wants to help, not someone who just wants us to like him or her; not someone who won't say what we need to hear. But how do we open up this kind of friendship? How do we stop hiding from ourselves? There are some steps we can take.

Find a real friend. Look around you and find someone of

your own sex that you respect and who is not competing with you at work or church or in your neighborhood. Someone who has nothing to gain by knowing the real person you are, except the joy of a deeper friendship itself.

Give permission to be truthful. Make a covenant with your friend that you will listen to the comments given about you. Ask for information that is not designed to make you feel good but information that will help you improve. Ask for information that will help you know better what you are doing wrong.

Pray for a spirit of truth. Both your friend and you need help to be truthful. We are programmed by our culture to be nice and that is good, up to a point. But honesty is better than just being nice. We are "nice" to our enemies. We need honesty. We need it because without God's help we aren't really honest.

Meet regularly. But watch out that your meetings don't become mutual admiration meetings. Put a definite limit on the meetings, such as an hour at a time and a period of 30 to 90 days, after which you can renew the covenant or make one with another person. Make a commitment to pray that you will listen to each other and that you will allow God to intervene each time you get together.

Keep in touch with your purpose. Remember that you are seeking to empty the three sins we have been exploring: (1) living up to our own ego ideal (2) giving ourselves orders and (3) stifling our real feelings. Bring along a Bible to help stay on course and read together a section that you both agree on. Ask yourself several questions, either privately or aloud:

How am I hiding from myself this week?
Whom have I been angry with lately?

Do I really love others in my own family as much as I want to?

Learn the freedom to be weak. Remember that no one is perfect, including you and your friend. Neither of you is the teacher. Both of you do things that are wrong, and you can learn how to be free, by talking over wrongs that need to be changed. If God has helped in the previous week, talk about it. But be wary of much talk of how good you have become so that it not become a recital of mutual goodness. That tends to become self-honoring and finally self-worshipping. First thing you know you've put the mask back on. Both men and women are proficient at making themselves look good. We are schooled that way all our lives. But way deep down inside we know we aren't. Only God is good. That point was underscored by Christ when he was with us. His comment bears looking into because it is such a stress-relieving truth.

In the books of Matthew and Luke there are clear guidelines for people who meet in truth covenants such as we have been describing. In Matthew 19 someone came to Jesus with this question, "Good sir, what good thing shall I do to inherit eternal life?" "Good?" he asked. "There is only one who is truly good—and that is God" (Author's paraphrase). Then Jesus went on to prescribe how a person can get to heaven, by referring to the Ten Commandments. He knew that it is an impossible achievement by ourselves. That's why God wants us to know we need him.

And in Luke 18 we read this powerful message: "Two men went to the temple to pray. One was a proud, self-righteous Pharisee, and the other a cheating tax collector. The proud Pharisee prayed this prayer: 'Thank God, I am not a sinner like everyone else, especially like that tax collector over there! For I never cheat, I don't commit adultery, I go without food twice a week, and I give God a tenth of everything I earn.' But the corrupt tax collector stood at a distance and dared not even lift his eyes to heaven as he prayed, but beat upon his chest in sorrow, exclaiming, 'God be merciful to me, a sinner'" (Luke 18:10-13 LB).

In this translation of the Living Bible Jesus adds the deep words we need to hear when we have been hiding from ourselves. "I tell you, this sinner, not the Pharisee, returned home forgiven! For the proud shall be humbled, but the humble shall be honored."

True friends help us to be humble. They don't trample on us. They don't compete with us. They don't tell us how good they are, thereby compelling us to tell them how good we are. True friends are honest with *themselves* as they are with us. Thus they help us to find the freedom to be weak.

If we are willing to be weak together, then he becomes strong in us. When two or three are gathered together in his strength, then he is in us. And he is our friend as well as our Lord. That's the offer that Jesus gave to us who are possessed with ourselves, walled off by ourselves, sufficient in ourselves. He says in John 15, ". . . You are my friends if you obey me. I no longer call you slaves, for a master doesn't confide in his slaves; now you are my friends, proved by the fact that I have told you everything the Father told me" (John 15:14,15 LB).

When we are caught in the stress of self-worship, Christ is an enemy in our eyes, of our own making, because *we* want to be king. But when we are willing to be honest with ourselves we can drop the heavy mask of ego stress that self-worship is. And Christ becomes our friend as we see the truth and obey him. It's almost as though Christ is asking us a question in the middle of our ego stress. "Are you hiding from yourself?" If so, you are carrying around a heavy load. But there is no need to. Why not try a truth covenant with someone you trust or you would like to learn to trust? God wouldn't mind being a part of it. In fact, he is the indispensable part.

Eight

Family Finances Will Get You if You Don't Watch Out

Dr. Louis Kopolow, staff psychiatrist with the National Institute of Mental Health, along with other colleagues over the years, has considered the emotional cost of the economy and its affect on you and me. Both optimism and pessimism are affected by the economy. Underlying fear and greed effects stock market changes every day. One government document states, "The change in the economy has created a feeling of insecurity, financial strain, and fear of the future."

But stress emerges from all the lurking corners of our minds, not only when we have too little money, but when we have too much money. A familiar line in a popular play that has run for years says it well, "Whether you are rich or poor it's nice to have money."

Stress is so pervasive in our lives. Harvey Brenner of the Johns Hopkins University, in Baltimore, Maryland, completed a study of psychiatric admissions in New York State covering 127 years. He and his associates discovered that admissions to psychiatric hospitals increased whenever our economic conditions turned downward. We know that money changes all of us, even the thought of getting or losing money arrests us. Dr. Brenner found that economic

stress causes a rise in alcoholism among working class
families, and a rise in suicide among families in higher
economic levels. He also found that males in the 45- to
60-age group are admitted to hospitals for emergency
treatment of emotional distress in subsequently higher
numbers during an economic downturn.

Unemployment takes its toll, not only because people
need money, but because people lose their social place in
the community, their sense of security and the prestige
they have learned to expect. "In the long term phase,"
according to Dr. Kopolow, "substantial unemployment or
belt tightening can produce strained family relationships. . . ."

What can a family do when economic stress becomes a
reality? Our changing economy has become such a difficult thing to foretell that the fear of the future which Dr.
Kopolow mentions is a recurring thing. It seems that
every few weeks there is a new report about a hoped-for
rise in the economy, followed by a prediction of a
downturn. One person put the stressful feeling that results from such uncertainty this way, "These days when
you see the light at the end of the tunnel, you have to be
careful. It might be a freight train."

Albert and Barbara Buono, who run a family restaurant
in an upstate New York village, explain the way they are
beating the economic pinch in their business. "Nothing
goes to waste," Barbara said. "That's what makes a restaurant work in a tight time." To beat the high cost of fuel
at home they installed a wood-burning furnace in their
basement that works in conjunction with their oil furnace.
By heating the water that is tapped off the regular furnace,
they cut their oil bills to practically nothing and they get

their wood free. "But that won't last," Barbara said. "We'll buy an inexpensive wood lot somewhere and we'll still beat the system."

Where you and I are concerned, economic stress boils down to family finances. Some people are licking the problem by turning to creative solutions. It beats just sitting around worrying. "It's amazing how little you can get along on when it's necessary," said Earnie Morrissey of Atlanta. "I learned that when I went back to college for my master's degree. We sold our house and cut our expenses to the bone. We planted a garden and canned what we couldn't eat." When Earnie told me about his success, he was clearly enthusiastic at beating the system. "There's a certain satisfaction in finding how little you can get along on," he said.

But the problem for most of us is that we let our family finances get out of hand. First thing we know we're on a treadmill. It's no longer a case of joy from beating the system. The system has the upper hand. The little snowball at the top of the hill has become a smothering giant as it rolls down the hill towards us. That's the stressful predicament we get into with family finances. But there is a way out.

Actually there are two ways out, and both of them should be used at the same time. One is, do all the simple but helpful things that will immediately change the family expense habits. Stop the flow of money or "profits" out the back door, as Al and Barbara Buono would say it. The other is look for the spiritual cause and set it straight. As far-fetched as that may seem, there is often a spiritual problem at the bottom of the mounting pile of unpaid family bills.

First, let's look at the immediate steps—the ones that shut the barn door before any more cows get out. Here are some clues that can put the family at work on the problem.

Get everyone involved. It's important to get family effort going, no matter how little our individual effort may appear to be at first. When we talked about this in our family, one of the boys asked, "Why, all of a sudden, do we want to save money?" The answer is, "Because that's the only way to start—suddenly." It's a little like Great Britain's decision to start driving on the right side of the road. You can't change over gradually or someone will be hurt going the wrong way. To avoid someone getting hurt, everybody's got to drive right. When a unified decision has been made concerning family finances, there is an immediate feeling of relief. "We're going to *do* something about it."

List your wants vs. your needs. Two columns on a sheet of paper are all that is needed to start. The idea is to get as many of the items listed on the "needs" side transferred to the "wants" side by asking, "Do I need it or just want it?" If it can be realistically seen as a want, it can be purchased later. "When is it necessary to have this? That's a helpful question when the budget is out of line. But if that becomes too restrictive each person can be allotted one or two "wants" with a dollar limit, and this can be relaxed when the family is out of the financial woods. All we are doing here is making our lifestyle fit our income.

Start in the kitchen. The policy here is symbolic and practical, too. The key again is decisiveness. It can even be fun to see how Al and Barbara Buono's kitchen plan can work in our own family restaurant. "Nothing goes out the kitchen that isn't used," say the Buonos. In a restaurant profitability starts in the kitchen, and it can start there in the family as well.

Watch your credit card use. Carry the cards you pay up each month, such as oil company cards, and put the others in a safe place at home. That helps cut down impulse buying; makes a person think twice before charging purchases at 18 percent per year (and more, when you consider that some balances run more than a year, and we pay out much more than 18 percent—even as high as 36 percent). Figure it out on your balances that drag on over a two-year period.

Close out all "interest only" loans. By lumping them together, if necessary, in one payment that reduces the principal each month, the savings will start mounting up right away. But shopping around for the lowest interest rate will be important.

Fix up the old car and recane the old chairs. Sometimes you can make this a game, too. If you can swallow your pride and drive an old car you can save the wear and tear on the pocket book. There is satisfaction in driving a Beetle 120,000 miles without an engine repair. And you can actually keep a car battery as long as 117,000 miles, by not having a car radio and keeping the car in the garage. It saves the strain on the battery during cold weather starts. I have one to prove it. It's still going strong and I'm proud of it.

But the old car is also just a symbol. Ever try to recane some old chairs instead of buying new ones? Call the furniture restorer about caning chairs. It's easier than you think. And there are lots of other symbols that can become dollar savings, too.

But what happens if we can't make our lifestyle fit our

income? If that becomes a desperate situation, there are some people in the community who can help. I wish I had known about them sooner, particularly when I counseled a compulsive buyer. She couldn't keep herself from buying things, and her master's degree in psychology only helped her know *why* she did it. It didn't help her stop. She bought because her parents pushed her out of their lives by giving her money. "Go buy something," their actions told her, and she did. As a compulsive buyer in adult life, she went to an attorney to consolidate her bills, but it didn't help. She didn't pay her attorney either! Finally, she found a group called *Buyers Anonymous*, and whenever she got the urge to buy, she would call one of the group for support. It helps to find someone who has licked the same problem. There are other versions of this group. The original was *Alcoholics Anonymous*, and there is another called *Gamblers Anonymous*. Each one operates on principles that have worked for years. Essentially, they are: (1) admitting you can't help yourself; (2) joining a group that knows how and wants to help; (3) taking each day at a time and keeping from buying (or gambling or drinking) *that* day; and, (4) helping someone else.

I talked with a New York cab driver about this one day on the way to the airport. "It worked for me," he said. "I owed $50,000 and most of that was owed to the illegal loan sharks who loaned at a rate of five dollars a week for every hundred I borrowed. Each week I paid the charge and never reduced the principal. I was in deep financial trouble, but I had to admit first that I was a compulsive gambler before I could be helped.

"You've got to know you are wrong," he said, "before you can change." There is a word for that. It's called confession. When that is followed by repentence and regular meetings with others who know they need one another, they lick the problem. It's much like getting religion.

The stress that comes from financial trouble can have a spiritual root, or a lack of it. Here are some of the underlying roots of financial distress:

Greed: Pretty tough label, isn't it? But we might as well call them as we see them. Acquiring more and more for ourselves—whether it is money or possessions—adds up to the same thing. Sometimes greed starts out by measuring the quality of life by the possessions we have. Two cars, a boat, a summer cottage, or a travel trailer are neither good nor bad. It's when we "need" them and can't afford them but we get them anyway that gets us in the end. Measurement of life by our possessions slips up on us unnoticed. The love of possessions or things is a root of distress.

Self-love: The reason love of possessions is wrong is that it is the way we get trapped into preoccupation with ourselves. Real love looks out for someone, wishes good for someone, gives to someone. But love of possessions is loving ourselves, taking care of us, wishing good for us, giving to us. A family where each one is acquiring something just for self is a bankrupt family, whether or not the money has run out. And it usually won't be long before the money runs out. If we truly love someone, we are willing to deny ourselves.

On a very personal level, Joan said to me one day, "The way I buy is important. I try to buy with my heart. And my prayer is, 'Lord, help me to buy right.'" That doesn't mean we are always spartan in our family, nor does it

mean we never blow the bankroll on something that is
fun. It does mean, when finances are limited, we need a
little help. The perspective that comes with Joan's prayer
is helping us, literally, to buy right.

Lack of priorities: Sometimes financial difficulties come
from lack of interest in the future. The old saying, "If you
don't know where you're going, any road will get you
there," has some truth in it. Up to a point. But most of us
do care, when we stop to think about it. Some advance
planning is necessary if we are to reduce financial stress in
the family, including financial stress that comes when the
person dies who is responsible for handling financial and
business details. The most difficult day in family life is
when death occurs, and that is complicated when nothing
is in order. Usually, one person has been handling the
family finances for years before death and the other members of the family are often lost financially as well as
emotionally. Once in a while it is good to let someone else
pay the bills, make bank deposits and check the bank
statements, just to let the family know that things are in
order—or how to get them in order.

Christian Resource Associates, of Orange, California,
distributes a personal estate planning guide that allows a
person to record the information that is needed in the
settling of your estate, regardless of how large or how
small. Their point is that such things should be done in an
orderly and less costly manner, to enable your heirs to
make realistic financial plans for the future. It's an intriguing and easy-to-follow set of worksheets to put down the
things the family needs to know concerning 25 separate
items. I have listed them because they provide a handy

check list for anyone who wants to put major family business items in order.

1. Wills
2. Family birth record
3. Family marriage record
4. Family military record
5. Personal employment record
6. Social security
7. Pensions
8. Safety deposit box
9. Real estate
10. Personal property
11. Bank savings and loan accounts
12. Investments
13. Money on loan
14. Debts
15. Life Insurance
16. Hospital, medical, accident insurance
17. Fire insurance
18. Automobile insurance
19. Tax information
20. Burial plans
21. Special requests
22. People and companies to be notified
23. General information
24. Location of valuables, papers and records
25. Procedure to follow at time of death

Putting life in order is what we are talking about. When we do that, responsibly, we feel less stressed and we show the ones we love that we care. But there is a major danger to be aware of here. If we allow what starts out to be responsibility to become an obsession with building up an estate, we will have missed the point of life. We will not only be shallow, we will live stressful lives, just trying to keep our estate intact, watching the stock market so closely, day by day, that we forget to enjoy the day itself. If we succeed in getting an estate of significance just to pass it on, we may even *cause* stressful living for our children when we are gone. Financial responsiblity is different from laying up treasures for our children. Jesus has something to say about that way of life. His words were directed to us. "Lay not up for yourselves treasures upon the earth . . ." (Matthew 6:19 KJV). But there is a sense in which the sin of laying up treasures carries over to the next generation. Once in a while it is important to look ahead, with the balanced perspective we get from imagining what our chldren will be preoccupied with. Suppose it were our own son, now grown, standing at the edge of the crowd listening to Jesus talk about life and priorities.

"Teacher," a man in the crowd said to him, "tell my brother to divide with me the property our father left us." Jesus answered him, "Man, who gave me the right to judge or divide the property between you two?" And he went on to say to them all: "Watch out, and guard yourselves from all kinds of greed; because a man's true life is not made up of the things he owns, no matter how rich he may be." Then Jesus told them this parable: "A rich man had land which bore good crops. He began to think to himself, 'I don't have a place to keep all my crops. What can I do? This is what I will do,' he told himself. 'I will tear my barns down and build bigger ones, where I will store the grain and all my other goods. Then I will say to myself, "Lucky man! You have all the good things you need for many years. Take life easy, eat, drink, and enjoy yourself!'' But God said to him, 'You fool! This very night you will have to give up your life; then who will get all these things you have kept for yourself?' And Jesus concluded, 'This is how it is with those who pile up riches for themselves, but are not rich in God's sight'' (Luke 12:13-21 TEV).

Either way, family finances will get us if we don't watch out. There are several causes of stress related to money: worry over not having enough, worry over losing what we have, worry over ways to make more, or just preoccupation with measuring life in terms of money.

The message of Jesus to those who are caught in the grip of financial worry is a simple one: ''Do not be worried, . . .'' he said. And then he asked one of the more profound questions in life, ''Which one of you can live a few more years by worrying about it?'' (Luke 12:25 TEV). What Jesus implied was that we can actually increase our financial and physical health at the same time.

Nine

Get Healthier as You Grow Older

We can literally lengthen our lives and increase our health, even in middle age. Most of us are only vaguely aware of this truth and when worrisome health problems occur, or when our physical capabilities begin to wane, we tend to forget it altogether. But it's true. We have a marked effect on our own health, not only in the way we live out our lives, but in our reaction to unexplained physical changes and the body ills that we know exist.

When my brother died of a heart attack at age 36, I began to think more seriously of my health and how I could live longer. I talked to a physician and he said, "The best way to avoid a heart attack is to have parents who have strong hearts and have lived a long time." He explained further, "There are things you can do, but a healthy heart is hereditary—and so is long life." What that doctor didn't know is that there are significant things we can do.

While Dr. Meyer Friedman and Dr. Ray Rosenman were developing the notions that led to their book, *Type A Behavior and Your Heart,* many doctors were not willing to consider stressful living as a cause of heart failure and death. Now that this has been generally established we are discovering that the impact of stressful living is far more widespread in our bodies than just our hearts. The list of stress diseases is already long, and growing. Some of the ailments include: gastric ulcers, hypertension, high blood pressure, cardiovascular disease, mental breakdown, migraine headaches, colitis and temporary diarrhea. Stress may even be linked with cancer, according to some. But whatever we may discover about the causes of illness in the next several years, we already know that authorities have labelled stress the worldwide number one health problem.

In the face of all this, it is literally possible to improve physically as we grow older and, within limits, extend our lives in several ways: through improved diet, "tailored" exercise, effective sleep habits and a common-sense approach to life stresses. The answer is partly contained in meditation and prayer—but not merely as a "super-ruminator," as Dr. Louis Kopolow of The National Institutes of Mental Health cautions. The answer is in using a number of approaches that we find right for ourselves. For instance, here's a practical clue for a simple headache caused by stress. When I was manager of a corporate management school near Washington, D. C., I used to develop a fuzzy headache at the end of a day of matching wits with very capable middle level managers from around the country. I didn't like to take aspirin, but I did respond to the jogging vogue that started in the middle '60s. I laid out a one-mile route around the conference center grounds and each night right after the session, I would get sweated up during a good run and then jump into a cool swimming pool. (Incidently, I found out later that jumping into a cool pool is something you shouldn't do. Sometimes the shock of cold water makes you gasp and take in a lung full of water and drown. It is a sure cure for stress but the cost is a bit steep.) The real headache remedy for me was strenuous physical activity. In 15 or 20 minutes a headache can actually be run away.

Out of experiences like these and my concern when my brother died, comes an understanding of some of the things that help us increase our health. When unhealthful stress mounts up, exercise can become a great relief valve, as long as we tailor it to our own individual needs and physical condition. It is also vital that we learn to enjoy the exercise itself rather than be pressured by it. There are two ways we can run up a flight of stairs, for instance, and both have to do with our state of mind. We can run to meet a schedule, fretful all the while, or we can forget time pressures and run for the enjoyment alone. It's the same with any exercise pattern.

But what about the worrisome illness or physical pain that occurs when we don't find an immediate answer for our ills? After a while worry itself will make us ill if nothing else does. And that alone can shorten our lives. When the nurse announced after my first company physical that my blood pressure was probably better than my son's, I was elated. But the physician later said, after looking over the charts, "There are one or two things you should know. You have a first degree heart block and the iron count in your blood is low." He tried to ease my mind by saying that the low iron count could be due to a faulty reading because of trouble they had noticed with the equipment. "And a first degree heart block is nothing to worry about," he added. "It just means that the electrical impulse takes two hundreths of a second longer to get through your heart." He went on, noticing my concern, "There is usually a little scar tissue that causes it. From an old illness, perhaps, or something as simple as a more recent virus."

It wasn't until I was walking back to my office that I began to be conscious of fear. It came on as though a monkey had suddenly plopped on my back. I had just crossed New York's Park Avenue. I felt somehow detached from all the people around me, because no one knew how temporary my life could be, I thought, and no one cared.

We have all known this fleeting worry about our health. It's when the fleeting worry becomes an overriding concern that we get into trouble. It's when we worry yet stay away from the doctor that we become as much the problem ourselves as the illness or discomfort. When I found out later that I could still exercise, eat anything I wanted, and not change my lifestyle, I realized a first degree heart block is just something you live with. There is such a thing as a healthful attitude toward illness, and it is an important part of actually growing healthy as we grow older. But that doesn't happen overnight, nor are we ever immune to health-worry.

Years later, when I developed a painful pricking sensation in my eyelids one morning, I thought nothing of it. But when the prickling persisted a few days and my skin began to dry up and flake around my eyes and on both sides of my nose, I began to worry. "What strange malady have I got now?" I wondered and off I went to the family doctor. He has a marvelous relaxed manner about him. He told me what the trouble was *not*, but I could see that he didn't know what it *was*. A few days later it spread to my forehead and I went to a skin specialist.

"It started out as a prickling feeling," I said, and he looked behind my ears and at my hair and said, confidently, "There's nothing to worry about." A good doctor seems to know that one of his main services to patients is to get them to stop worrying. "You're just using the wrong shampoo," he said. "What you've got is seborrheic dermatitis." If he'd have said the name of my mysterious malady first, he would have added to my suspense and my growing anxiety, but having first said, "It's the wrong shampoo," he treated my worry before he treated my skin problem. "Try this kind of shampoo," he said, "and here's some cream for your face and a prescription for your eyelids. Come back in a week and your face will likely þe cleared up."

"But why do I have this all of a sudden?"

"I don't know. You've just got it. But it will go away if you treat it."

It wasn't until later that I found even skin trouble can be caused by stress. Sometimes a visit to the doctor is worth it, just to hear him say, "This is all you've got wrong with you. Otherwise you're disgustingly healthy."

Health-worry is one of the biggest enemies of our physical condition, especially as we grow older. In that sense it is possible to kick the worry habit and grow healthier as we grow older. Dr. Robert Orr, a friend of mine who has a successful medical practice said, "I can't tell you the exact numbers, but I would say that well over half of my patients have stress-induced illnesses." And over the years I have reviewed a number of employee situations with industrial physicians who confirm the major role that stress and worry play in everyday illnesses. It is becoming more and more clear that a healthful attitude towards illness will help reduce it and this same attitude toward aging will actually increase your length of life.

Think for a moment about the impact of our general attitude about young people and old people. Across the United States I have asked audiences their opinions about these questions:

1. Whom do you feel most Americans would say are more creative: young people or old people?

2. Where do you feel ego (the belief in ourselves, and how capable we are) is the strongest among Americans: in old people or young people?

3. Which group of people do you feel Americans believe to be smartest: old people or young people?

For three years I asked audiences for a show of hands on these questions. In all, there were thousands people, generally ranging from their early thirties to the late fifties, with most in their forties. I saw a slow change in the three years from most people saying "The young are most creative. They are strongest in ego and smartest." But that changed to a mixed reaction, where the numbers voting in favor of young and old roughly balanced out. Over the next few years I expect to see this change to a perception that old people are *more* creative, stronger in ego, and smarter. Our national mood about aging is changing, but slowly. The reason this will be important is that successful aging and healthful attitudes toward ourselves as we get older are woven together—and will make up the fabric of our future health as individuals. The important point for us as individuals is what do *we* think? Or, more important still, what are we doing about growing more healthy as we get older?

Our health attitude is helped by doing some symbolic

things. Some of us have found a way to get rid of the habit of eating a massive amount of sugar, for instance. I avoid foods that list sugar first, second or third in the ingredients, and compensate with plenty of raw fruit. Also I found that a better quality of protein exists in some food than others.

As for exercise, we have found that a few, brief exercises in the morning provide a good mental setting-up that carries over into other activities during the day. If we miss in the morning, a simple set of exercises at noon are good for us (right on the office floor, for instance. But one day my secretary almost fell over me and I decided to shut the door!)

At night I take my dog Honey Lee out for a jog; she becomes so excited about jogging that I find it hard to let her down. We enjoy jogging *together,* under the stars, as opposed to my feeling I have to jog just for my health.

Out of these experiences I find some simple steps we can take.

• Pay attention to the literature on nutritious foods. Eat more dairy, fish and vegetable protein and less meat. Get some roughage in the diet. Eat less, as a general rule, and even fast (go without eating) once in a while to let the system become purified.

• Adopt a personal exercise program that gets you out doors more regularly, where you can get a spiritual uplift and you aren't beating the clock. Checking in with your personal physician is an important part of this. Then, if you can't get into the exercise habit by yourself, get your dog or your spouse or your children to run or swim or exercise with you. But remember, you are doing it for fun and for relationship as well as for your body.

• Forget the notion that we decline in ability as we get older and replace it with the more healthful realization that we *change* in our abilities. While the body ultimately wears out, making some strenuous exercises impossible, there are some other ways of exercising. One ninety-year-old woman said of a seventy-year-old man who had a cane, "When he got that silly cane, he took ten years off his life."

What we are talking about is learning how to be in the prime of life at our present age, rather than accepting someone else's notion of what is prime. There are some career activities in which we are at our prime in later life. Take a judge, for instance. Who would want to appear before a 12-year-old judge after doing something really wrong? Judgment and wisdom come from mistakes made and observed that we learn from. Give me an older judge who has really learned much from life.

Expectations are a key to capability in both the young and the old. The Pygmalion concept was tested years ago in a California school system where they took a number of bright children and changed their school records to show they weren't bright (and told the teachers that the children weren't bright). They took another group of "not bright" children and changed the records to show they were bright (and told the teachers they were bright). After an extensive test period, they found enough instances of different school marks and changed ability that they concluded that capabilities, at least in many instances, are a product of the expectations of the people around us. The same applies when we get older. One of our deeper problems in the United States has been the expectation that creativity and productivity peak out at age 65. But it is becoming more clear that this may be merely the result of the Social Security Act, drafted in the 1930's by people in their mid-30's who picked 65 at random as a reasonable retirement age. Out of that decision has come our current stereotype of the successful business person who retires to Florida, rises early in the morning to watch the sun rise from a Fort Lauderdale park bench or porch, then drives to Naples, Florida in the afternoon to watch the sun set. What a waste! But that's a picture of the lifeless retirement expectation we have generated in the United States. It has caused great frustration and stress—and the early deaths of otherwise healthy people. If we think we are supposed to die at retirement we increase the likelihood that we will.

What about durability of life? Can we actually live longer based upon our way of living? Some studies indicate that we can, even beyond the Type A and Type B studies performed by Drs. Friedman and Rosenman.

The management literature used to say that managers had more illnesses and didn't live as long as people in other occupations. Then the literature changed somewhat and observed that *middle level* managers seemed to get ulcers more than top level managers. Whenever I mention this to a group of management people, I usually add, "Top level managers don't get ulcers as often. They are just 'carriers.'" And there usually is a ripple of appreciation around the room. But the point is that whatever walk of life we are in—bricklayer or electrician or secretary—we can be more healthy and live longer if we are meaningfully employed. It's not whether we are on top. If our work is useful and we know it, and others around us know it too, we'll likely live healthier and longer lives than if we really aren't needed—or if it doesn't make a real difference if we are gone. Durability of life depends at least in part on meaningfulness, and even on reputation to some degree. But there are even further considerations.

People seem to live longer in certain areas of the world than in others, and that appears to be a combination of climate, economic level and cultural respect for old people, to name a few factors. A relatively high number of old people live in certain parts of Russia, such as the Caucasus Mountains and in the Ecuadoran Andes. "So who wants to move there?" we ask. But take a closer look. In the areas just mentioned there is a frugal but nutritional diet, a high degree of physical activity for the elderly, and an appreciation of the wisdom and economic contribution of old people. Further, there is often very little change in life style where people live longest.

There is a relational cause of longer life, too. A German sociologist reported that married people live longer. To which some wit might reply, "It only *seems* longer." The point is that people who love and trust each other, such as those who are *happily* married, actually do live longer! Good health comes from lives that are lived not so much for self as from those that are lived selflessly. Paying attention to diet and exercise and rest is important. But when we add to this the ability to stop being anxious about our own existence, we are on the right track. This upward-outward view toward our lives is worded differently in the book of Proverbs, Chapter 3:

". . . let your heart keep my commandments; for length of days and years of life, and peace they will add to you. Do not let kindness and truth leave you; bind them around your neck, write them on the tablet of your heart. So you will find favor and good repute in the sight of God and man" (Proverbs 3:1-4 NASB). And later, following more spiritual advice, Solomon adds, ". . . It will be healing to your body and refreshment to your bones" (Verse 8).

Refreshment, healing and years of life are spiritual gifts given by God to those who are discerning. They are not reserved for a select few. They are natural gifts enjoyed by the Methuselahs who were described in the books of the Old Testament.

Since then we have forgotten how to live long and productive lives because we have taken to worrying ourselves to death. The underlying answer to becoming more healthy and living longer is the kind of relationship that eliminates worry over ourselves. "Be not anxious" is healing advice from the Great Physician. By acting on it we can actually become healthier as we go through our hectic pace of life.

Ten

Beating the Pace of Life

How many times have you heard or said, "I never seem to have enough time anymore," or "I meant to get started on that, but I never have the time." Often what we are really saying is, "I never really decided that I wanted to do it in the first place."

Often the pace of life that crowds in on our lives is really a lack of decisiveness. During most of our lives we allow someone else to set the priorities of life for us, and often the priorities aren't very meaningful.

Our daily activities can be lumped quite easily into four categories: work, fun, meetings and travel. And all four categories are packed tightly into our busy lives. Even our fun is accomplished on a schedule, so that our day looks something like this:

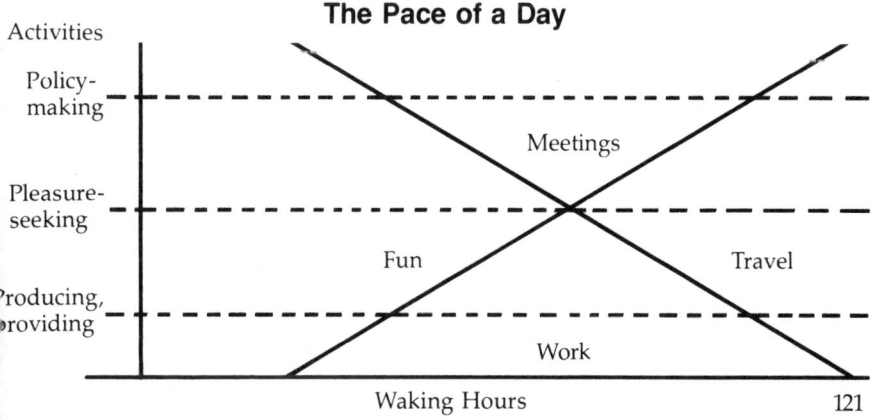

The Pace of a Day

• Workers spend their days having a little fun, a lot of *work* and little travel.

• Policy-makers spend their days having a little fun, a lot of *meetings* and a little travel.

• Pleasure-seekers would like to spend their days in fun and travel.

This lighthearted look at the pace of life can apply to people who work at home as well as away. But the people I have described as pleasure-seekers, who would like to spend their days in fun and travel, end up as frustrated as anyone else. Because even fun and travel can get wearing and purposeless. A dear friend of ours from the Washington, D.C. area, jokingly says she feels her grave should have this inscription: "She always seemed to be busy but never seemed to accomplish anything."

The opposite of accomplishment is absenteeism. It is one of the symptoms of stressful living. Not just the Monday morning or Friday afternoon or Sunday variety that can easily be seen on company, school or church absence records. Most of us absent ourselves from the personal things we say we need to get done but never get around to, because we are avoiding them. This is *personal absenteeism*, and it is as chronic a problem as the industrial kind that can more readily be checked. Here are four questions that can help us check ourselves and relieve the stress of the pace of life:

1. Is it possible to do all the things I am trying to do in the time I have?

2. Why am I trying to do the things I have set out to do?

3. Are the things I am doing worth doing? (Enjoyable, profitable, meaningful?)

4. What do I really want to do but never seem to get around to doing?

Sometimes, in looking at the things we do in our tightly packed lives, we realize the pace of life is getting to us. It's as though we are just going through the motions of enjoying life, the way some people travel through Europe or the United States on a whirlwind vacation. The If-this-is-Tuesday-it-must-be-Belgium joke is more funny if you aren't totally wiped out by the pace of the trip.

We found ourselves "oohing" over the rim of the Grand Canyon a few years ago on a family vacation trip. Our schedule was so hectic that we never got down to the floor of the Canyon to feel it from inside. It was almost like the cartoon of the vacationing family being shooed back into the family station wagon by the father who said, "Hurry up. You can see the rest of the view in our home movies."

The modern pace of life is stamped firmly on our vacation itineraries on both sides of the ocean. When Joan and I were in London on a quick side trip—sandwiched between speaking engagements in Europe—we decided to spend our time as profitably as we could between sightseeing and shopping, with a little British theater thrown in. We managed to squeeze in two Agatha Christie mysteries during the evenings, and such places like the Tower of London in the daytime. We peeked through the gates at Buckingham Palace, walked around the Dome of St. Paul's, worshiped in Westminister Abbey, shopped at Selfridges, and were on our way to Windsor Castle when we realized we had not yet changed our tickets for re-routing to Amsterdam. That should have done it as far as Windsor Castle was concerned, but I refused to believe we couldn't do both—until I began to see there's only so much hurrying you can do with a wife who refuses to walk at a race step through London. Joan said, with some despair, "It's not possible to do all this and enjoy it, too." "Oh, no," I said, "There's a chance we can fit it all in," and I even walked ahead to try and speed her up.

We finally reached the ticket office after several near misses, down the wrong streets and in wrong directions. By then I had a very dim view of the adequacy of London's street signs and its numbering system. When it was finally our turn to talk to the airline's reservation agent I announced that we wanted to redirect our flights and that we also were trying to get to Windsor Castle within the hour. This approach had worked so often in the United States that I had assumed it would work as well in London. But it seems no one can move a ticket agent through the complexity of international recomputation of fares, routes, and plans in ten minutes. "In thirty minutes, sir," she said, looking at me calmly.

"Thirty?"

"Yes, thirty. Or more."

I sat fuming as politely as I could in the plush chairs. But Joan was quietly waiting beside me, enjoying the forced relaxation while I was fighting it.

"OK," I said, finally, looking at her. "Let's have lunch somewhere and forget Windsor Castle."

By the time we got to a nearby restaurant, the Lord had spoken to me quietly but powerfully. "You're trying to enjoy too much," it seemed to me he was saying. I leaned over the table to Joan then and said, "Forgive me for what I have been doing to us."

The pace of "enjoyment" is mostly *our* pace, and that can turn good times into stressful times. But it is like that when we aren't on vacation, too.

Joan has settled into the weekday life of a wife who "does not work." She teaches piano, takes courses at a nearby university, assists in the church rummage store, takes voice lessons, attends choir practice, participates in two midweek programs at the church and a neighborhood Bible study. And she runs a home that is "too big for the family," she says. She told me one of her secrets of getting through the day when she overschedules. "When there are too many things to do and not enough time, I ask God to help me by saying, 'what do *you* want me to do today?'"

"It helps," she says.

"But remember," I say, with some jealousy, "you don't have to do all the things you do. You can stop doing most of them whenever you want." This is true of most of us. The answer to the question, "Is it possible to do all the things I am trying to do in the time I have?" is wrapped up in the next one, "Why am I trying?" And there the age-old ego question comes up again.

If the things we are trying to do are mostly ego trips in disguise, then we are doing too much. Ego is useful. Ego trips are not. Not if we are filling our lives with ego trips, because our love affair with self is getting out of hand. And there is no question that all of us are in love with ourselves. To say otherwise is hypocritical. The Apostle Paul had a comment about that. "No man despises his own flesh." And Jesus referred to our love affair with ourselves when he said, we ought to "love our neighbors as ourselves." If self love becomes a kingdom of self and is expressed in most of the things we do, then we are doing more than is good for us. And the pressure of life mounts up. Are the things we do worth doing if they only add to our life pressure?

What is worth doing? What is enjoyable? What is profitable? What is meaningful? These questions can be answered only by us as individuals, but our answer is better given as we reflect on the words of the Apostle Paul to the Philippians, ". . . Whatsoever things are true, whatsoever things are honest, whatsoever things are just, whatsoever things are pure, whatsoever things are lovely, whatsoever things are of good report; if there be any virtue, and if there be any praise, think on these things" (Philippians 4:8 KJV).

Our prayer can be, "Lord, what are the true, honest, just, pure, lovely things you want me to do in my life today?" This prayer, spoken sincerely from an open heart, can cause us to think on these things in a practical way and help us to answer the question, "What is worth doing?"

The fourth question is a test question. "What do I really want to do but never seem to get around to doing?" If we are living committed lives, rather than self-centered lives, we will not want to do only things for ourselves. There are surely *some* things we will want to do for ourselves, but there won't be a number of things we want for ourselves that will disregard the well-being of others in our lives. Not if we really examine our wants with others in mind.

Here is a way to examine our wants:
1. List three to five things you really want at this point in your life.
2. Draw a line under the last one, then ask yourself, "If I get these things, will I be happy?"
3. Now write down any additional wants that come to mind. (Likely, more will come.)
4. For each one, write the impact on others in your life when you receive or do the things you have said you

want. Ask yourself, "Will the impact be good on the other people in my life?"

5. Last, write down the impact *on your own life* of the things you want to do. Now that you have thought it over, will these things be good for you and others?

These five steps in determining what we really want can help us set priorities in the midst of our hectic pace of life. And priorities help.

Another way to beat the pace of life is to learn how to relax for brief periods in the middle of the day, particularly at lunchtime, and at the end of the day when we are able to gear down. It is surprising that such an apparently simple thing as relaxing takes a little training in order to really do it. Have you found it difficult lately to turn off the engine? To really change your pace?

Here are 10 simple steps to follow in relaxing. They don't require transcendental meditation in the eastern, mystical sense; they are just practical ways to relax the body, mind and spirit. In some cases it works better to have someone read these steps aloud while you follow them.

RELAXATION EXERCISE

1. Sit comfortably in a chair with both feet on the floor and your hands resting on your knees or on the arms of the chair.
2. Roll your eyes up as though you are looking above and behind your head. Then close your eyes as you keep them rolled up. (This gets your attention off whatever you have been thinking about, because it is an unusual position for your eyes.)
3. Focus your attention, now, on your right hand, and

imagine that a balloon is tied to the middle finger and is lifting it up.

4. Let your hand rise as the balloon lifts it. It doesn't matter how high, but it is a sign of relaxation if your hand is well off your knee and in the air.

5. Imagine you are now walking on the beach. You can feel the warm sand shifting as you walk. You can see the waves spraying in the air. You can even hear the tumbling of the waves as you walk along.

6. Now the sun is setting colorfully and you see a small boat coming toward the beach. As it touches the shore a person steps out and comes to you.

7. A concern or problem or interest has been forming in your mind and now you tell the person what it is. The person listens and you have a better idea of what you should do.

8. Now you recognize that the person is a messenger from God and you are ready to say anything you want. You can ask for help or be thankful, or just appreciate his presence without saying anything. And you can listen—more clearly. There is no need to hurry.

9. Now you are ready to leave your imaginary beach and to let your hand come down. When you are ready, you can open your eyes and speak. It is likely that you will feel the time has been good for you because you have been able to relax and think about things that were on your mind.

10. You are wide awake now and ready to go about your day.

You can do this ten-step relaxation-prayer exercise as many times as you wish without detriment because you are the one in charge. And as a more relaxed person, you can pray more freely during this time. What you are really doing is allowing yourself to come away from your everyday world into a time of simple quietness, or into a relationship with God. This is a practical way to follow the Bible instructions to "Be still and know that I am God." It can work, with practice, and become a time of deep physical and spiritual refreshment.

An even simpler way to do this is to awake a little earlier in the morning and, after a long, hot shower, lie on the bedroom or bathroom floor and relax. You can pray or meditate as long as you like, because this is your private time. Chances are you won't fall asleep because you are on the floor, and this is a way of telling yourself (your body specifically) that you are just relaxing instead of intending to go back to sleep. If that doesn't work, set your alarm.

The answer to the problem of pace of life can be helped by techniques such as these, but we need to be careful not to assume that we can handle the pace all by ourselves. Whether we use one of the techniques above or some other technique, the important point is that we need to ask ourselves once in a while whether even our techniques are filling up our lives.

We can profit from asking God to help us not be kidded into thinking we are in complete control. We need a way to check in with God. Joan's question works for her. "What do you want me to do today, Lord?" is a question that can help clear our hearts and minds. But the question isn't to be asked just once for each day. It is available as many times a day as we become pressed in by nerve-jangling schedules of time or the perplexity of unclear priorities. It's such a beautifully simple way of keeping in touch.

These are ways of beating the pace of life, but there is still another way and that is to learn to say no. Even a "no" to so-called good things is wise at times. Say no to committee meetings, association offices, even church responsibilities. When we examine the pace of our lives, we often find we are doing too many things—good or bad—for not good reasons. Consider the lilies," Christ said. "They toil not, neither do they spin. . . ." Jesus knew that the pace of life gets too much sometimes, and he knew how to get away from it.

"But how do we do that when we don't have time to get away?" we ask.

The answer is something like my father used to say about money. "It doesn't matter how much money you make. It matters what you *do* with the money you make." It's the same way with time. All of us have enough time. Everyone has 24 hours in a day. And we can get away from our version of the pace of life by saying to our Lord, or to someone else we care about, "I have enough time— for you, and for me." Otherwise our own personal world can be a very lonely place.

Eleven

Loneliness, Fear and Celebration

Some people are lonely and don't even know it. Others know it, but don't know what to do about it.

Loneliness is no respecter of persons. It afflicts the rich and the poor, the old and the young, the farmer and the city apartment dweller. None of us wants it. Few of us are prepared for it.

Loneliness is nothing like aloneness. It has nothing to do with how many people are around. Getting away to be alone is one of the privileges we all enjoy, whether we prefer fishing along a mountain stream, walking beside the ocean, still-hunting for deer, or shopping alone on a crowded avenue. Aloneness is something we seek, at times. It can help resolve our stress. But loneliness resolves nothing. Extreme loneliness causes some to become prostitutes, and others to take their lives—some quickly by suicide, and some slowly, like a widow. The tragedy is that there are enough people in the world so no one needs to be lonely, yet some people are lonely a good share of their lives. Is it because we choose loneliness?

After giving a talk on loneliness, I asked a group to give me any additional thoughts on the subject. A woman said, "I have been lonely at times, and people have come to help, but I wanted them to go away. I wanted to be lonely." I didn't understand what she was saying until later on when I thought about my own experience. When my brother died suddenly of a heart attack at Christmastime, I needed to get away. Nobody could help me at that time. I needed to question God in a very private dialogue. Somehow I knew that no one else could give me the answers to my questions—not a member of my family, not a minister, not anyone. A few days later when the Christmas parties started, I thought I was ready to go to one, but when I got there I couldn't go in, and I stayed outside in the car thinking of the impermanence of Christmas parties. Slowly, I entered into a communion with God in a new way. But it wasn't loneliness that I had sought. It was the opposite. I needed spiritual communion. The choosing of loneliness that people sometimes experience is not so much that they want to be lonely as it is a willingness to accept loneliness, if necessary, to gain something more important at the time—such as new insight or awareness of reality or closeness to God.

Loneliness happens at different times in a person's life and it often causes stress to the people who are looking on. When my oldest son Kevin ran away at 15, he left a note on the dresser that said, "I've got to run away and I don't want you to try to find me. There are some things I've got to straighten out and *nobody can help me.*" Those words cut deep into Joan and me because we suddenly realized our son had become lonely while living right beside us, and we hadn't known it. We had been directing a Junior High youth group at our church because we felt our sons needed the nourishment of others in the Christian way, but our popularity in the program separated us from our two older sons instead of bringing us closer. Part of the reason was that the youth group became our toy and a good share of our love was going out to the group, while not enough was going out to our sons. Kevin's note said, "I'll call you every day to let you know that I'm all right." So we prayed for wisdom and every day when Kevin called, we said, "We're not going to try to find you, Kev, as long as we know you're all right. When you're ready to come home, we want you to know that this is *your* place. And Kev . . . we love you."

The next Saturday morning Kevin came home. It happened while I was in the garage, trying to cope with our loss. The overhead garage door opened, and I looked at him standing there with his hand still on the opened door, looking at me, tentatively. I knew I could have blown everything then. All I could do was say, "Welcome home, son." Then I began to let the Lord teach me how to show Kevin that I really did love him.

One of the principal solutions to loneliness is love—the kind that perseveres and learns to accept different feelings of someone else, whether or not we understand the cause. Love keeps the door open when things aren't going well, so a deeper relationship can develop.

It's important to show a welcoming attitude to a person who makes an attempt to bridge a gap. Hurt feelings in relationships develop into long-term separation and loneliness when tentative attempts at reconciliation aren't noticed or are ignored. When Kevin came home he might have left again if we had pounced on him or shown that we were hurt more than happy when he returned.

One family that we know has a different kind of separation problem whenever there is a family reunion. Two of the aunts haven't spoken to each other for 20 years or more. So, whenever a reunion rolls around, someone in the family makes sure that Aunt Theresa doesn't sit at the same table as Aunt Carrie. And the rest of the family suffers.

Another family was affected by the stress of a strained relationship between a man and a woman who had been married for years. The whole thing blew up one day when Bill didn't answer a question from Mabel. He had been reading his paper as usual and didn't hear her question. Mabel harped a bit on it, and Bill snapped, "Mabel, if you don't stop, I'm going to leave." Mabel said, "If you walk out that door, you'll never get back in." "Oh yeah?" Bill replied, threw down his paper, and walked out. An hour or so later, when he had cooled down enough to return to the apartment, the door was locked. Bill never got back in. The fact that Bill and Mabel acted that way is all the more tragic when you realize they were grandparents. They lived the next ten years of life apart, and caused years of stressful living for their children. When Bill died years later, Mabel went to his funeral and a year later she died, quietly, of no apparent cause—except, perhaps, loneliness. Loneliness shortens life. It slowly robs a person of the desire to live.

Years ago, a German sociologist studied longevity of life and found that married people live longer. In discussing this finding with groups around the United States, I often hear the same light-hearted response I mentioned earlier, "Life just *seems* longer when you're married."

One successful executive—we'll call him Kent— commutes over an hour to work and arrives home just in time for a hurried supper. By then the children are tired and cranky, and by the end of the supper time his wife, Ginny, has reached the end of her patience. As soon as the children are in bed, Ginny heads for the television set, not caring what's on, and Kent sits in another room reading the paper. Sound familiar? This could be the first sign of one of those marriages that just *seems* longer. In a few years we might as well call them Bill and Mabel. There are a lot of lonely marriages like this. Most get that way before couples realize what's happening. Some couples hang on to lonely marriages for years. But divorce or separation is not necessarily the answer. That can cause even more loneliness.

A practical solution to loneliness is to learn how to keep our everyday conversations vital and real. That helps keep the relationship alive. The question is, how do you start after you have lapsed into the habit of not communicating? Joan said to me one evening, "Let's have a conversation tonight." I said, "A conversation?"

"You know what I mean," she said. "I say something. Then you say something." "Oh," I said, and we broke up, laughing over what has now become our adopted joke about the difficulty of real dialogue. After a pause she said, "You first." That's another of our little games, but it points up an underlying secret of conversation. It doesn't matter who goes first or how you go about conversation as long as you *both* decide you want to talk.

Talk is an antidote to stress. But there is a difference in quality of talk. Real conversation is a solution to loneliness. But real talk isn't easy for everyone. It can be squelched so easily when one word strikes the wrong chord or when it turns to harping like Mabel talking *at* Bill. Talking at someone encourages withdrawal and loneliness.

While writing the manuscript for a previous book, I began to withdraw from Joan. It was a bad habit I had begun to learn. So I suggested to Joan that we go to New York City for an overnight stay in a hotel. Just the two of

us. As we were leaving our hotel to go to a movie, Joan did
a very wise thing. She said, "I have the feeling I am not as
important to you as I once was." I thought about that. It
was such an arresting way to open a conversation. She
hadn't said, "You are doing me wrong." She hadn't ac-
cused me of anything, but I could feel her concern. It was
her *feeling* she was expressing, not an accusation. That is
one of the keys to rebuilding a relationship. She had
begun to feel lonely, and now I began to feel her loneliness. We went to a little crepe place on Third Avenue after
the movie and talked for a long time. Then we decided to
walk back to our hotel so we could talk some more. We
even stopped on several street corners when we got en-
grossed in our dialogue, and finally we came to our hotel,
still in conversation. We were still talking at 3:00 A.M. in
our hotel room. We were learning again how not to be
lonely.

Here are a few ways to get un-lonely:

Try disconnecting the television set and storing it for one
month. One of the biggest drawbacks to dialogue is the
escape box that television often becomes. After a month, if
you decide to bring it back, put stringent rules on the use
of television in your home. Make the rules arbitrary and
stick to them. If there is some other escape device affecting
your dialogue in the family, no matter how harmless or
healthy it may be, toss it over the side for a month, with
vigor.

Learn to discuss your feelings without being judgmental.
Here is one way to put into practice Christ's commandment, "Judge not that ye be not judged." Judgment is the
parent of more judgments, and the grandparent of bitter-

ness. Bitterness is one root-cause of a special kind of loneliness that sometimes takes years to cure. In-laws often have a special problem with judgment and it spreads to other members of the family. In the early years of her son's marriage, Audrey and her daughter-in-law Ann had a breakdown in relationship that caused Audrey and her son Jim not to speak for 30 years. Now, Audrey is a grandmother in name only. She is in her late eighties. Her son Jim and Ann are in their sixties, and the grandchildren only now are beginning to realize the rich heritage of relationship they have been missing—and they see the unnecessary loneliness of their parents and grandmother.

Discover the freeing power of asking for forgiveness. A major step in relieving the tension of a hurt relationship is gaining the ability to say, truthfully, "I was wrong and I'm sorry. Please forgive me." Even if the other person can't yet forgive us, we become more free by confessing that we were wrong. Confessing our faults to each other is a prescription for dialogue St. Paul meant for us to apply to our relationships in the family as well as in a congregation.

Unlock your loneliness by forgiving before you're asked. Even if the person who has hurt you *hasn't* asked you to forgive him, you can do it anyway. Forgiveness takes only one person. And forgiveness is a way to renew our internal relationship, because *we* are renewed by forgiving someone else. There is a special self-made loneliness that comes from harboring an unforgiving spirit. Years ago I harbored a bitter feeling against a landlady who had kept my security deposit unfairly. Then I remembered some advice from my father who had said I should forgive a person even if he didn't know I was forgiving him—and I found a strange new freedom when I forgave my landlady.

We are forgiven (relieved of guilt, set free from *our own bonds*) if we forgive. Christ said, "If you will not forgive, you will not be forgiven." Those words rank with the most powerful of all the words of Jesus.

Recognize that the only truly lonely people are those who choose to be lonely. Sometimes it's better to choose loneliness if our spiritual well-being is at stake. But loneliness is a heart attitude as much as it is anything else. Living in loneliness can actually be a sin if it keeps us from the love and fellowship of Christ, who has offered fellowship to all of us, including the lonely.

Loneliness neither gives nor receives love. Love is the everlasting gift that God has provided us to overcome loneliness. In the beginning God was concerned over Adam's loneliness and created Eve. Today he has provided a way out of loneliness but it's not necessarily another Eve. Today he is saying, "How about a different relationship—with me?"

There are many results of loneliness. All of them are harmful. Take fear for instance—it's very close to loneliness. Often the two go together. When Joan and I were married, she was 17 and I was 21. We got married then because I was about to go overseas and I thought I would be able to take her with me. One week after we were married, I caught the train back to the Air Force Base, expecting I would see her again as soon as I found a place for us to live overseas. But that never worked out because the Communist guerillas in the Philippine Islands made life risky for anyone to live off base. For the next 17 months we were separated and very lonely. And there were times that I was afraid, when I saw all the love-letter marriages around me breaking apart. One after another, Dear-John letters came from wives and sweethearts who couldn't take the loneliness. But our letters kept reinforcing our love, compensating for the loneliness, looking ahead to the time we would be together again. Loneliness at Christmastime in the Philippines was overcome by plans for next Christmas. Fear that something could go wrong was overcome by trust that we wouldn't let things go wrong. Loneliness and fear are conquerable if we fix our attention on another day ahead when things will be different.

After 17 months of learning how to cope with loneliness and fear, I boarded a troopship for California and home, but I was yet to experience a new level of fear. A few hours out of San Francisco, we hit a heavy fog bank and the captain announced that the fog horn would be blown periodically to warn other ships. "Don't be alarmed," he said over the loudspeaker. "It's just a precaution." But a few minutes later, the captain's voice came on again. "Men. Stand clear of the water-tight compartment doors. We're going to close them and I don't want anyone hurt." We all knew why he was closing the doors. In case we were rammed in the fog only those in the rammed compartments would drown.

I strapped on my life vest as casually as I could, to maintain the mask of sophistication, all the while feeling a heavy fear deep down inside as I looked around me at the empty compartment. When I reached the top of the gangway, I saw that the entire deck was filled with men, from the front to the back and side to side. We were all there, looking in the same direction for some little speck of light on the California shore. And we all had our life vests on.

Finally, we began to see pinpoints of light that slowly became lines of light and at last the outline of the Golden Gate Bridge. The men way up front let out a cheer as the bow of the ship slid under the bridge. Then the cheer swelled as the middle of the ship slipped past. From side to side, the cheer became a roar and I was caught up in it as I watched the bridge slide over us on the fantail. We had come out of the loneliness of the inky Pacific, through the fear of what the fog might conceal, into a wild *celebration*.

True celebration never happens when we are obsessed by fear, nor when we are enshrouded by loneliness. When loneliness and fear are left behind, *celebration* is possible. Sometime in our lives there must be room for celebration. Celebration is the special antidote to the stress of loneliness and fear. We are made so that we can survive loneliness and fear, and it helps when we look ahead to a promise of safe harbor. For even the most lonely and the most fearful there is a promise of safe harbor in the covenant of Christ: "I go to prepare a place for you that where I am there you may be also." He said that after he had come to understand loneliness and fear and had overcome them.

When we live a life that is preoccupied with loneliness and fear, we are living crippled lives. A lonely or fearful life is not a part of God's plans for us. These crippling stresses of life keep us from living life in celebration. This is nowhere more clear than in the angels' announcement of Christ's coming to the shepherds who were living in the fields, keeping watch over the flocks at night. A shepherd's job is a lonely one, especially in the middle of the night when others are taking their turn at sleeping. When the angel appeared in the brilliant, sudden glory of God, it made the shepherds so filled with fear that they couldn't hear the real message. That's why the angels' first words announcing Christ's birth to the shepherd's were almost a commandment, "Fear not!"

Why did God announce the coming of Christ to shepherds at a lonely time and a lonely place, rather than at noon in the marketplace? Perhaps because the message is particularly welcome to lonely people who have been caught in life-work that seems unimportant. The reasons for the loneliness the shepherds felt were immediately removed when the excitement of God came down and the heavenly family was on hand. But that alone didn't help the shepherds, nor does it help us today if our loneliness is only replaced with awe. Only when the shepherds listened to the words of the Lord and abandoned their lonely way and their fear of this new wonder did they begin to know what celebration was. As they went to see the Christ, they caught the enthusiasm that God had and went with haste, running, stumbling, picking each other up, until they finally came to the place where they could see that the word of the Lord had already become flesh, and was dwelling among them.

When I relfected on this at Christmastime, driving home to our house in Pound Ridge one day, I realized that I had been lonely a number of times. Especially at middle age when I had learned, wrongfully, to value life in terms of achievement at work. I had come to judge life success by the number or articles I had written, speeches I had made and rewards I had received, rather than the relationship of love I had given and received. I did something then that I would find difficult to say in some groups because I had been wearing an invisible mask of self-protection that hid my loneliness. *Even I didn't know I was lonely.* When I saw this in my life, suddenly, like the shepherds, I was overcome with excitement and gratitude for the gift of his presence. I could hardly see the road then, because my eyes were filled with a very wet gratitude. "Thank you, Lord," I breathed with a hurt in my throat, "For coming to me in my loneliness—even when I didn't know." The rest of the way home I experienced a new celebration as I abandoned my loneliness.

If we are living lonely or fearful lives there is no need to. "Don't be afraid," is one of the most ringing messages in the Gospel. God has provided a Good Shepherd for all of us—even the loneliest and most frightened. I went straight home and shared this good news with Joan, because Christ had set me free from another self-inflicted bondage and replaced it with celebration.

Twelve

Get Out of the Success Trap

Working for one of the more successful companies in the world, with roughly 300,000 employees and $18 billion of revenue per year at one point in the company's history, I found it comforting that one of the questions asked by IBM's main line marketing division was: "What Is Success?" This question was asked in a program called "Perspectives," a school for high potential employees, who hadn't yet reached management and perhaps didn't want to. The point was made in this program that success is an individual thing that should be considered with career, family and personal interest in balance. When one of these interests gets out of balance, we lose our perspective and the dis-ease of "success-stress" begins.

The question, "What is success? is an important one for all of us today. All of us are reaching for success in something, whether we are a homemaker trying to nurture a family while considering some way to establish an identity, or a college student trying to obtain the right degree, or a person about to retire who doesn't know how to face the next several years. Just the question itself, "What is success?" reminds us of the probing thoughts of Socrates who said, "Know thyself," or the Jewish Scholar, Hillel, when he asked, "If I am not for myself, who will be? If I am only for myself, what am I?" These are arresting questions for people who are success-oriented.

Sometimes it helps to look at success from the vantage point of retirement. Sitting at the same table one day with Gil Jones, the second most influential person in the IBM company before his retirement, I asked him if he would be willing to give me his ideas on stress, now that he had just retired. Gill Jones had just completed a long and successful career, ending as the Chairman of the board of IBM World Trade Corporation, and member of IBM's Corporate Management Committee, among a string of other accomplishments. He looked at me closely. "Have you got twenty minutes that you would like to spend with me in my office?" It was an hour and a half later before we finished our talk and by then Gil Jones had outlined several things about stress and success. "Within three months after my first management job I had an ulcer," he said. "I learned over the years that understanding the cause is very important. You need an outlet, too, like exercise or some way to leave your work at the office. My outlet is squash," he added. "But stress comes back at different times throughout life, regardless of exercise and it can beat you down. Mental illness is a universal trait, and I've found that inward-looking alone will kill you if you do it long enough.

"What about all the successful retirees in Fort Lauderdale?" I asked, "Stress catches up with a person whenever he or she plateaus," he said, "and it really can catch up with you when you retire. You think even more about yourself then. You can get into considerable trouble by moving to a ghetto for retired people. They actually manufacture stress in retirement ghettos, you know. I think especially in the rich retirement ghettos where the people have lived a life of achievement and suddenly find their lives afford none of the success opportunities they had before." He looked at me closely. "I know a retirement ghetto where you are ostracized if you don't invite everyone in the community to your parties. If you are late at the golf course, your house guest must pay five dollars to ride in your own golf wagon. It's rules like these and plenty more that cause some retired people who are rich to live in a very small world."

That's what success can come down to when we pursue it to the exclusion of the rest of life. Success itself becomes an exclusive ghetto that really can become a prison of self-made rules.

The problems of success that Gil Jones and others have examined start long before retirement. Listen to Anne B, a former model, who told me about her success race. "I was two years old when my mother died. I was the second youngest of five girls. I had to take the role of mother at eleven when my older sisters went away to school. I remember even in Kindergarten I wanted to do better than anyone else in whatever I did. I graduated from school with honors and went into modeling. While enjoying a very successful modeling career, I held part-time secretarial positions to prepare myself for a business career after modeling. I demanded perfection from myself and finally made it to management. But stress was always a part of my life. My doctor warned me to slow down, but I allowed total involvement in my career to blind me to the signs that things were closing in on me. Then the physical breakdown happened, just when I was about on top. I had just one more step before reaching my goal. I remember being terribly disappointed in myself . . ."

Being disappointed in ourselves is a very real cause of stress and it doesn't go away easily. Anne had pulled out of a stress filled life after a long rest, but was ready to make another run for the top when I saw her one day at her desk in a California office. We talked about the things that are important in life and Anne began to listen more closely to God's direction. "I was looking too hard," she said in a letter later on. "I had to stop and give myself completely to him before I could realize why it is that I am here on this earth." There are times like this when we realize that we aren't supposed to live for success and we begin to ask, "where does the drive for success begin?"

Success begins with the desire to do something important or rewarding. Somewhere during age 21 to 35, people are more willing to work 10 to 16 hours a day for success. The more problems they can handle during those years the more opportunity they have to be successful later on. But the desire to be successful doesn't stop *when* we become successful. It is replaced by the desire to protect our success or to become even more successful. During a career school I held in New York, a capable engineer we will call Steve thought about success for several days. He came to me and the rest of the class with this question written on a sheet of paper, "To do something . . . what?" Steve had listed five attitudes that described his success search during his beginning career years. He said at first he had been idealistic, then frustrated, then defiant, then resigned, and finally, aware of what was important to him. It worked this way. When Steve joined his company, he thought he could become one of the stars in the corporation in short order, but after awhile he realized the company had hired a lot of other would-be stars and he became frustrated. When he wasn't recognized for his special level of worth as he saw it, he began to look for another company that would recognize him and got a job offer with another firm at three thousand dollars more a year. But his employer said, "If you'll stay with us we'll make it worth your while in the long run." He stayed and received more money but didn't get the sense of worthwhileness he was looking for. Then he became resigned to the likelihood that he might not become the star he wanted to be, and his resignation to this became apathy rather than content. That's one of the major problems of business—employees who have resigned but haven't told their companies.

There is a fine line between contentedness and apathy and most of us don't know when we cross it. But apathy can be a negative result of the stressful struggle against the competition in our success race. There are two additional attitudes that we should consider that can help free us from concern over competition. They are beyond the five of Steve, the young engineer who brought his attitude list to the career class. They are decisiveness and commitment. These two attitudes can help us deal with our stress.

Here's how our success trip often looks from an attitude standpoint, whether our success is career oriented or centered on our marriage.

SEVEN ATTITUDES THAT AFFECT SUCCESS IN LIFE

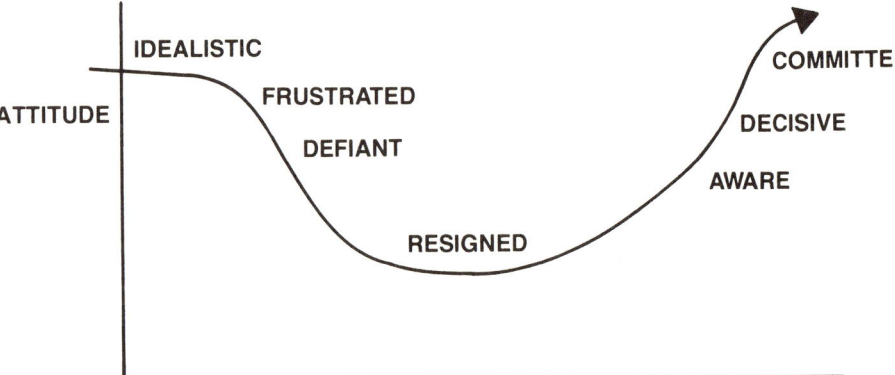

IDEALISTIC

COMMITTED

ATTITUDE

FRUSTRATED

DECISIVE

DEFIANT

AWARE

RESIGNED

This little map of seven attitudes can help us look at our own success trip and ask, "where am I right now in my career? Where am I right now in my marriage and personal life?"

What we need at several times in our journey to become successful is some way to look at where we are heading. A map of what has happened to others sometimes helps us look at the course we really want to take rather than the course we are on. The real question behind the one Steve raised, "To do something . . . what?" is "To be someone . . . who?" This question of personal identity has been clarified by a person named Erik H. Erikson who developed a life cycle that looks something like this:

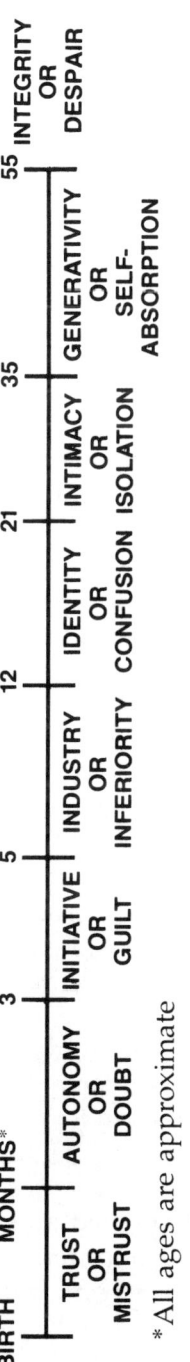

BIRTH

TRUST
OR
MISTRUST

18
MONTHS*

AUTONOMY
OR
DOUBT

AGE
3

INITIATIVE
OR
GUILT

AGE
5

INDUSTRY
OR
INFERIORITY

AGE
12

IDENTITY
OR
CONFUSION

AGE
21

INTIMACY
OR
ISOLATION

AGE
35

GENERATIVITY
OR
SELF-
ABSORPTION

AGE
55

INTEGRITY
OR
DESPAIR

*All ages are approximate

The beginning of this life cycle can be compared with Sigmund Freud's stages of early development often called oral, anal, phallic, latent, and adolesecent, but we need not go into those to look at where we are now or where we are going. The point is that a lot of people have gone through the success struggle at different levels and ages.

The people mentioned before, Anne and Steve and Gil Jones, have experienced parts of the same roadmap we are now on, with the same identity crises we may be experiencing right now. Some successful people have fallen into a few traps along the way, and others have gone around them.

Successful living is a matter of gaining maturity and wisdom more than getting a promotion or a new house. We get into trouble when we look at success with the tunnel vision that often sets in somewhere around age 21 to 35. It takes a lot of energy to hack our way through the jungle of uncertainty during these years, and most of our uncertainty is about ourselves and how good we are or can be. Personal worthwhileness is one of the underlying questions we all struggle with throughout our lives. And there is real pressure to succeed in order to get our income high enough to be self-supporting then family supporting in the style that our culture has influenced us to reach for. That's when the beginning of isolation can start and intimacy can be dulled.

After giving a talk in Toronto, I listened to a young successful executive who came to me and said, "I'm worried. I've been reaching out for success and I'm afraid I'm losing the ability to love my family." I thought I saw the tell-tale look of isolation in his eyes. When people become totally achievement oriented and lose intimacy in their lives they pay a steep price for success.

There is a special age crisis that often occurs around age 35, when a person realizes that life isn't going to be the achievement oriented success he or she had in mind. The "oh no! I'm not going to make it" feeling that crashes in on a person who has bound up all of life in achievement is sometimes too much to handle. The mid-thirties are often a time of self-absorption such as this but can be a time of generating deeper relationships with others.

Somewhere around 55 years of age is the point that Erikson labels "integrity versus despair." If health fails or our children despise us or our spouse runs away, or life has been all work and we are forced into early retirement—or if all of these happen—we become a candidate for despair. But it doesn't have to be that way. It is true that a 55 year old likely will have more health problems than a younger person and any other stresses that are added to that concern can become too heavy. And if a person has put in a 12 hour day for the past 10 years he or she is really out on a limb when someone says, "We don't need you any longer." But we need to remember that the choice between despair and integrity is exactly that—a choice.

Success traps aren't the malady of organizational people alone, nor are they the exclusive concern of people in middle age. They are the pitfalls of anyone at any level and any age who loses perspective. Success can be fun. It certainly isn't wrong in itself. "There's actually something called exciting stress, Don," said a 55 year old person who had regained perspective and was about to retire. "Age 55 is a very good age," he said. He had just told me of a little real estate business he had decided to retire to.

A friend of mine from Jacksonville, another Don Osgood, wrote to me and described stress from his viewpoint, after early retirement caused by a heart attack. "A roller coaster ride is stressful," he said, "but exciting fun for some, although not for me anymore. The closing moment of a big sale is stressful, just before the prospect becomes a buyer, but it is thrilling to a professional salesman. But when I let stress get out of hand in my life, it becomes anxiety, and that is what did me in for awhile." Success by itself isn't wrong at all. It is only wrong when we let it get out of hand.

What goes wrong with success? What makes success turn sour? One major cause seems to be narcissism. Not the face in the mirror variety but ego narcissism. Listen to clinical psychologist Sheldon Bach. "You used to see people coming in with handwashing compulsions, phobias and familiar neuroses," he said during a magazine interview. "Now you see mostly narcissists." In the same article, social critic Tom Wolfe called the 70s the "me decade"—the "doing my thing" decade. But we can find people at various ages who have managed to put their finger on life success without a me-first attitude. Don't look for internationally famous people, necessarily. Listen to Bob Warner who enjoys normal success and happiness without a national reputation. "I've got as much reason to be stressful as anyone else," he said, sitting in an office at IBM's Executive Development Center on Long Island. "For me, it's easier to prevent stress or to reduce its effects before it can do any real harm. I do this through a regular physical fitness program. Exercise, coupled with a Christian attitude of service, allows me to maintain a balanced approach to success as I see it.

When we look at the kind of stress that comes with success, we begin to see that success and stress are woven together, but some people have worked out a way that allows inner peace in the middle of the stress that success

brings. Some actually thrive on it. Then how do we stay
out of the success trap and still be successful? Part of the
answer was spelled out by Dr. Nate Adams, Pastor of
Stanwich Congregational, a small New England church
that serves people who live in Greenwich, Stamford, and
Westchester County communities near New York City.
But Dr. Adam's words apply to people living in any community and in any workplace.

"Work is not to become the center of our life," he said
one Sunday morning. "That is not God's plan. Most people try to find their worth in their work. But God is saying
to us that our worth is in our relationship with him.
Ambition is, in part, proving to everyone else how important we are. We don't need to prove who we are by what
we do. Christians don't need to spend their lives in office
politics. We don't need to run a race that no one has asked
us to run. Worth is a gift of God."

The notion that we don't need to achieve anything to be
worthy people in God's sight is a freeing one, when we
stop to think about it. We don't need to live up to someone
else's expectations for us of success. Nor do we need to
live up to our own expectations of success. But this idea is
hard to understand in our minds alone. What we need is a
heart message that speaks specifically about success and
there is one strong, clear heart message about this in the
fifth chapter of the book of Romans. The beginning of that
chapter is especially meaningful in our consideration of
success as paraphrased by Ken Taylor in the Living Bible,
"So now, since we have been made right in God's sight by
faith in his promises, we can have real peace with him
because of what Jesus Christ our Lord has done for us. For
because of our faith, he has brought us into this place of
highest privilege where we now stand, and we confident-

ly and joyfully look forward to actually becoming all that God has had in mind for us to be."

These words have a number of messages for us, especially if we reread them prayerfully and ask for the message we need to know, way down deep. Then things begin to come together for us in the middle of our wondering about success. When we realize that God has had in mind something for us, not he will have something in mind, but he *has had it in mind* for a long time, perhaps from the moment of our birth—then we begin to get a glimmer of what our success can be. If we can get our ego ideal out of the way and find what his ideal is for us, we will live the most freeing way of life there is. Then we will be at peace in our success, whatever that is for us, as we confidently, joyfully look forward to actually becoming someone real, rather than being obsessed with achieving something important. It is this quest that God resolves for us, and it is one of the most freeing realizations in life to finally know that we can't break out of the trap that success can be by ourselves.

But before we can really look forward to becoming what God wants us to be, we are required to do something else, and in that Gil Jones of IBM appears to agree with a very sound Christian concept, although he didn't say so specifically. When I finished my discussion with Gil Jones about stress and success, he looked me closely in the eye and said, "Don't look back. If you worry about the past, your life is going to be miserable. The happiest people are those who look to the future." Jesus' message is, "You don't need to look back. Look at me and I will let you see yourself as you are and as you can be."

A new kind of success is just around the corner. That's what we will be looking at in the final section—growing in, not up. And we won't be worrying about our childhood hangups or our ability to determine our psychological state of being, or even how big we can become. What we will do is look at the deeper level of freedom that lies in relationship. We are about to go right to the heart of the personal stress issue and find a simple, workable way of life with an upbeat note all of us can share. And the chances are we will.

Part Three

Finding New Freedom From Stress

Thirteen

Breaking Out of Prison

The reason the word "freedom" is so alluring to us is that we spend most of our lives in prison. We live with the illusion of freedom much of our lives. We fashion our own private prisons in the same way we build walls to protect us, stone by stone. And one day we become walled in without knowing it. Stressful living is the result of that.

In Part II we looked at circumstances and relationships that, in a sense, often put us in prison and cause us to live stressful lives. And there are other pressures and other prisons that we have to deal with as well. But when we finally deal with each pressure point in our lives will we then be free? What if we try all the secular stress cures we know? Will we then be truly free? Let's look more closely at this.

There are several specific stress management approaches we can take right where we are, in the middle of our circumstances. Here are five of the most often mentioned ways to break down the walls of overstress that can plague us. Each approach has a special value—and a particular pitfall, if trusted too much. We will look at them in a general way and then consider each one more deeply.

FIVE BASIC APPROACHES TO MANAGING STRESS

- ANALYTICAL
  (Goal clarification, problem-solving, "straight thinking")
- ATHLETIC
  (Exercise, diet control, proper rest)
- AWARENESS
  (Bio-rhythm, bio-feedback)
- ALTERED-AWARENESS
  (Meditation, yoga, relaxation-response)
- ATTITUDE
  (Personal relationship improvement)

The analytical approach is a "western" way to deal with stress that we might expect a business person or a scientist to use. It includes thinking about the goals in life that are really important and trying to determine in advance a way that the important things won't be crowded out by the urgent but less important things. There are several ways to do this. One is simply to write three or four life and career goals on a sheet of paper and think about them for awhile, similar to the way described in the chapter, *Beating the Pace of Life.* Next you can consider realistically when you want to reach your goals and how they might be accomplished. Then, after giving some thought to them, imagine you have already achieved each one. Now ask yourself, "What do I want, now that I have achieved the life goals I have listed?"

When we do this we often find that a deeper life goal comes to mind. We experience a releasing of our minds from the immediate or surface goals so that still deeper desires come to the surface.

By writing out several personal goals for all of life and ranking them in order of importance we begin to lay the groundwork for solving future problems and for setting even today's priorities in better perspective. When these life goals are discussed with the family so that the goals of each person are considered, we begin to find that a goal-clarifying, problem-solving approach can help us overcome some of the stress of uncertainty in our lives.

Day-to-day problem-solving techniques also help release us from stress. One way to do this is to spend more time in identifying what the problem is before trying to solve it. Problem *identifying* is the single most important part of solving any of life's problems. By getting into the habit of asking ourselves, before putting our solution into effect, "What is the real problem here?" We can save ourselves a lot of stressful solutions that just don't work for *our* problem. One of the most effective class sessions I have used in a new manager school is a problem-solving workshop, where groups of five or six people examine the people relationship problems submitted by each person attending—without trying to solve them. Participants are asked continually to raise the question, "What's the real problem here?" We have found that there is an almost universal increase in comfort just by identifying the problem and discovering that others have similar problems.

These analytical or straight-thinking approaches reduce today's stress and help us anticipate potential stress. But dependence on this alone doesn't resolve stressful living. That is clear when we think of the many analytical people who have developed a stressful "Type A" reaction over a period of time.

The athletic approach has been increasingly popular. For years we have been aware that a balanced diet, regular exercise that works up body heat, and a consistent pattern of sleep can actually maintain resistance to stress. With a doctor's approval, a person of any age can benefit from hard physical play or work, providing it is regular enough and we have prepared our body for it. Exercise and diet control actually increase our energy level and provide immediate, temporary relief from stress. But there is a danger of overlooking the real cause of our stress if we assume that the athletic approach is the only technique we need. If our stress is caused by a loss of relationship for instance, jogging isn't going to resolve the problem. It's just going to make us feel good for a time.

The awareness approach helps us when we don't even know we are under stress. We have trained ourselves to meet difficulties so well that often we don't even know there is increased pressure within us. That is why bio-feedback has become helpful to some. Bio-feedback is the term for several techniques of recognizing little clues from our bodies that tell us when we are under excessive stress—when our minds are still at work convincing us that everything is normal. Some people use electrical devices that sense a change in blood pressure and heart activity during certain kinds of work, activity or relaxation. This is done to get used to noticing what it feels like when they are really relaxed. It helps to learn the things that are really relaxing as opposed to stress-producing. For instance, golf can be very stressful even though most people play it to relax. For all its popularity some people feel golf is just another way to destroy a good walk!

Bio-rhythm is the term used by many for charting their

own life rhythm. It is based upon a personal pattern of ups and downs that seem to follow roughly a 30-day cycle for both women and men. People who follow this approach closely will chart their "on-days" and "off-days" for months ahead and plan their important appointments accordingly. For those who like this approach, both bio-rhythm and bio-feedback provide a basis for daily stress adjustment. And there are some impressive reports of improved safety records where people are asked to use extra caution during their off days. But there is a danger of a self-fulfilling prophecy here, and awareness alone doesn't resolve stressful living.

The altered-awareness approaches, including yoga, transcendental meditation, and the relaxation response, have been used for centuries in one form or other. Dr. Benson's relaxation response (a non-religious mental relaxation technique) was widely publicized after the eastern mystical approach of transcendental meditation gained western publicity. Generally, these approaches produce mind-over-body relaxation that can be used anywhere, but these don't provide the final answer either. There is a danger of denying reality or of blunting reality when we retreat into a form of meditative isolation that often results from altered-awareness. And eastern approaches, even though supposedly not religious, can lead people down a non-Christian path.

The attitude approach, or personal relationship improvement, touches one of the major causes of stress: loss of relationship. By reaching out to others in an attitude of sharing and commitment there is release from stressful living. *Stress-releasing, dependent* relationships rise from trusting someone, and this can be a major solution to stressful living. But the danger exists of over-dependency on unreliable acquaintances or even dear friends who cannot meet our needs for strength or counsel when we most need it.

There are many practical ways to deal with stress. The five we have just considered can be restated even more simply as follows:

Five Practical Steps to Personal Stress Management.

- Discover your own stress level.
- Choose your own goals in life.
- Balance your diet, exercise and sleep patterns.
- Develop honest, caring relationships.
- Get in tune with your real purpose.

These basic solutions to stressful living have been around for years, yet for all their practical application, stressful living goes on. That is because breaking out of the prison of *stressful living* (as opposed to selecting different approaches to managing stress) is very tricky business. Most of us spend a good share of our lives breaking *into* new prisons of stressful living. Adam and Eve's story is our story. Being out of relationship is a prison itself. And that is what can happen when we start breaking out of whatever prison we are in without some spiritual perspective. The modern day notion that we've got to get our head together by ourselves misses the point. If we get it all together, what have we got? Maybe a lost relationship. The conclusion? There is still a better way.

There is a radical idea around that is so foreign to our human way of thinking that we can't seem to see it. But it carries the possibility of a whole new realization of freedom. It's not a new idea, as most profound ideas are not, but there is telling evidence that it has worked for years.

We are to find new freedom from stressful living within the circumstances and relationships that we think are prisons. We are not to duck them or throw them away hoping to find freedom by indiscriminately ridding ourselves of our marriage or job or personal concerns—whatever they are. Sometimes we should get rid of such problems, but that shouldn't be our first solution. Not without tapping into the possibility of becoming new within ourselves. There is a universe inside us waiting to be discovered. To do that we've got to be able to see freedom from stressful living with a spiritual insight that isn't discernible with our eyes. Without that kind of openness—not just to see or hear but to *know* something new—we will rumble right on by freedom at 80 miles an hour. When the Broadway musical, "Shenandoah," opened, it soon had a hit song about freedom that said, "You can't get to freedom on a train. Freedom is a full time occupation. Freedom is a state of mind." That's getting closer to the discovery of freedom from stressful living. But we're still not quite there, as long as we think of freedom as a mind process alone, or a selection of stress management techniques.

Anything dealing with the mind has to do with being in control. Anything dealing with the heart has to do with being out of control. Our minds like to be independent, but our hearts don't like independence at all. We get closer to knowing freedom when we are open to the outrageous idea that being *out* of control is freedom. And that is where we begin to see the prison of self-interest more clearly. In learning how to be free of the shackles of self-interest and self-dependence, we are on the right track.

Let me explain that further. On a speaking trip to Stockholm, Paris and Nice, I decided to visit Copenhagen on the way over and Madrid on the way back, just to see two cities I had not visited before. Joan said to me, "You're filling up your schedule so full that you're going to be tired out." She remembered our trip a year before when I dragged her through London, trying to pack in more than the trip would allow. "I wish you would just go direct to Stockholm and get some rest and come home after Nice," she said. I couldn't see why two more cities would hurt, but Joan reminded me of the way I drive myself on a trip and said, "You need to get out of control. Have you prayed about your schedule?" I hadn't prayed enough, I guess, because the two days just prior to leaving had been filled with rushing off to Washington and Long Island, and now I felt some added tension from this unresolved issue with Joan.

When I finally prayed, "You take charge of the decision about the two extra cities, Lord," I suddenly realized that I had been too wrapped up in what *I* wanted. I realized, too, that it was important to Joan that I accept her concern, whether I saw things the same way or not. I realized, also, that if she were going to Europe and I wanted her to come home a day sooner, just because I wanted her home more, I would be hurt if she were not willing to do it. When I told her I was willing to accept her wish for my trip, I felt a new release. I had let go of my control of my schedule, already packed full, and showed Joan, and God, that I was willing not to be in control. That helped me the next day when I couldn't be in control—when my flight was canceled and I had to go to London instead.

It helped me again when I learned the London Air Traffic Controllers were on strike and we would have to wait for hours on the ground before flying on to Stockholm by way of Copenhagen. I had wanted to see Copenhagen, but I was allowed only to look at the outside of Copenhagen's airport. When we landed there were two clear announcements by the flight attendant, "Passengers who are going on to Stockholm are *not* to get off the plane." I thought, "God really knows how to teach a person to relinquish control. I can't even get off the plane!" But I sat looking out at Copenhagen's airport without a bit of uneasiness at not seeing a famous tourist city. The reason I wasn't bothered was I was out of my mind. I don't mean I was crazy. I was at rest in the sure knowledge that I was pleasing Joan instead of me, and saving myself from an overworked week. I was out of my mind because I was in a different heart attitude. I was free to *not* go to Copenhagen.

Freedom is a heart attitude that keeps us from self-interest, and deepens our relationships. Self-interest is the slavery that we spend most of our life trying to break into, and we work ourselves into stressful living that way. The prison of self comes from trying to be in control of everything. "If we can just get our head together . . ." is one of the big lies we have believed. But sometimes God makes us a prisoner on a plane, or in some circumstance in life, to teach us how to be free inside. And that turns out to be the only real freedom there is.

This new inside freedom is not a new idea at all. It's a profound idea that has been experienced down through the centuries by some famous people such as St. Paul, one of history's real prisoners whose freedom became more real as he spent time in a real prison. He wrote a letter about that to the Christians in the City of Philippi: "Everyone around here, including all the soldiers over at the barracks, knows that I am in chains simply because I am a Christian. And because of my imprisonment many of the Christians here seem to have lost their fear of chains!" (Philippians 1:13, 14 LB). In the next chapter Paul gives us some clues to finding inward freedom that can be helpful in many of our circumstances today.

Ten Clues to Inward Freedom
from a Prisoner Named Paul

1. Don't fight the prison you are in. If you've got to be a prisoner, be a willing prisoner.
2. Overflow with love, but grow in knowledge and insight at the same time.
3. See clearly the difference between right and wrong. Be inwardly clean.
4. Live in eager expectation.
5. Stand beside each other with one strong purpose. Be willing both to trust and to suffer.
6. Don't live to make a good impression on others.
7. Don't just think about your own affairs. Be interested in others and what they are doing.
8. Don't demand or cling to your rights. Stay away from complaining or arguing.
9. Stop worrying about your own plans.
10. Help each other.

When we look over the clues that Paul has passed along to us from prison, we begin to see different kinds of freedom for the times when we can't change the outward circumstances of our lives, or the times when we shouldn't even try.

Let's take another look at ourselves. We look quite different from the triangle that behaviorist Abraham Maslow drew when he said we have a series of graduated needs. (See Appendix.) He was right in that, but he didn't list the needs in quite the way we see them when we think of inward freedom—and he might even have missed a need or two. Maslow said our strongest need is a physiological one, followed by a need for security, then love, then ego integration and finally, self-actualization. This last one seems not only out of place, but wrong, in the Christian context. It is a picture of a person trying to see how big or good or complete he can be *in his own strength*.

The Apostle Paul said something very different from that. When he was in prison he didn't say, "I'm being kept from what I'm supposed to be." He said, in effect, "I'm supposed to be right here. Now and then, I'm struggling with being here, but I know this is where I am supposed to be. I need someone to be a brother to me, but I don't need to be self-actualized anymore than I am right now. What I need is to be God-actualized." He became free not by trying to be somewhere else but by accepting his circumstances. Paul was learning that some times in life we are to release more, relax more and yield more, even in prison.

In our overemphasis on self-growth, we sometimes develop a stressful outer shell that imprisons our inner self, because we strive constantly to be somewhere else or someone else. What we need is not so much to become someone, but to *be* someone, right where we are. In his strength, not in ours. That is what God has offered to us.

When the Apostle Paul had been running around Israel trying to get control of the Christians, because in his head he thought they were wrong, he was finally brought to a burning bush and confronted with reality. When God spoke to him it was in a direct way, something like this:

"Why are you fighting me, Paul? You are the wrong one, not the Christians!" In the next several weeks, Paul became a real person. He recognized his true identity—("I'm the wrong one!") and was forgiven. He had reached a level of new identity and forgiveness.

We can't really accept forgiveness until we recognize that we are wrong. We can't be forgiven until someone is willing to forgive us. And we must *accept* forgiveness, if we are really to be forgiven. When those three steps happened in Paul's life, he was ready to go to a new level of inner freedom.

Forgiveness is one of our most profound needs. *More profound than self-actualization.* When we accept forgiveness from someone we become a receiving person. Then we know we can't get everything all together by ourselves. When we *accept* freedom we are set free from our past, at the moment we accept it. If we still feel guilty for the past, we are not free. The message of Christ is that God is ready to set us free from guilt. He says, "You are no longer guilty, if you can accept my forgiveness."

One of the most stressful things in life is trying to live up to our notion of what it means to be good or great. The Christian message to stressful people is that God wants to liberate us from the destructiveness of that kind of pressure. But real freedom comes from being willing to open up the hidden areas of our lives. Paul had been living a destructive life. He was on the road to self-actualization by presuming to help God out, without getting his orders first. And that's what a lot of us do these days in our attempt to be religious on our own. It's almost as though Paul was told, "You're on the wrong road, Paul; what are you going to do about that?" Now and then that's the same question God asks of us.

The freedom to have real relationship comes when we recognize our true identity or direction with respect to someone else. A person without a real relationship is a person in prison. A husband and wife that are living in a superficial, hidden marriage are in prison. That's one reason why marriage hasn't been working lately, even in cases where both husband and wife are Christians who believe in the sanctity of marriage. Relationship and commitment go together. And we can't have commitment without giving up at least some of *our* way for the benefit of someone else.

When I gave up Copenhagen, I told Joan by my action that I was committed to her wish more than my wish. And I received a strengthened relationship. When we give our "rights" away to someone who cares about us, we become free of our rights. Free people don't spend much time looking out for their rights anyway. Did you ever see a really free person who always demands his own way?

Take another look at Paul several years after the burning bush. He even said to the people in Philippi that he was a slave of Jesus Christ. Does that sound like freedom? Not to the superficial self. Not to the person living in anxious struggle. But the committed or giving person will say, "Yes. That's freedom. Freedom from me. When I give myself for someone else, I'm free of my own trip." That's why it wasn't a complaint at all when Paul said, "I'm a slave." He used to be a slave to Paul, and now, speaking to the people in Philippi, he was saying, "I'm a willing prisoner even here in jail, because I am doing God's will."

Down through history we get revealing glimpses of what man's real motivation is, once he understands where he's going. In the old European monarchies the desire of subjects to serve their king to the death, if necessary, is evidence that men and women want to follow a true leader or cause. That notion has changed some in our current world, but the inner desire to find the true leader or cause is still very much with all of us. It is often buried way down deep so that not everyone recognizes it. It is a desire for a real relationship with someone who knows where *we* are going. In that relationship there is a new kind of freedom from ourselves.

In the play, "Shenandoah," a young black boy says to his master after the Civil War has set him free, "It ain't easy being a slave boy. It takes practice!" In our own personal Civil War, we have been practicing being a prisoner most of our lives. Now it's time to practice being free. That is what we must now deal with even if we think we are free!

Fourteen

So You Think You Are Free!

Personal freedom has several levels. A little freedom of spirit often reveals a hint of deeper freedom yet to be realized. The reason freedom is so universally searched for is that it has been planted in our hearts as something to be discovered. We literally have been called to freedom.

In the words of J. B. Phillips' *New Testament in Modern English*, "The whole creation is on tiptoe to see the wonderful sight of the sons of God coming into their own. The world of creation cannot as yet see reality, not because it chooses to be blind but because in God's purpose it has been so limited. Yet it has been given hope. And the hope is that in the end, the whole of created life will be rescued from the tyranny of change and decay and have its share in the magnificent liberty which can only belong to the children of God" (Romans 8).

This "magnificent liberty" is not merely an opportunity for us to gratify our lower natures but an opportunity to look into the source of freedom that is available to us. The limitation we face is that we get a little freedom and think we have the whole gift. This is another of life's big lies that we believe. But there is a bottomless well of freedom literally reserved for us by God himself. Every once in a while someone breaks through our superficial layer of living and helps us see this.

Between the years 1090 and 1153 there was a powerful yet loving French Christian named Bernard of Clairvaux. He was an insightful priest who could sway an audience with deep notions about identity, love and God. Behind these notions lies the possibility of new freedom from stressful living.

When I heard of Bernard of Clairvaux in a quiet breakfast discussion held by an Episcopal priest named Robert Dresser I felt some of the spiritual rustling down inside that Bernard must have felt. Bob Dresser's simple explanation of Bernard's four phases of love sent me home thinking that we spend virtually all of our life not knowing what is really going on in our relationship with God. We don't see the four phases because we seldom get out of the first one or two. The four phases are: loving self for self's sake, loving God for self's sake, loving God for God's sake, and loving self for God's sake.

To understand any of these we need to realize that we find true freedom in life through love, rather than self-examination or psychology alone. That road hasn't really led us out of the wilderness of stressful living. Rather, we have fallen into a sort of analysis paralysis. We have worshipped psychology as our high priest rather than using the information from psychology as something that may or may not work in our particular circumstance. The primary way out of our paralysis of introspection is through the primary relationship between God and self. Let's explore this as deeply as we can.

In the process of maturing we move from one to the

other of Bernard's stages, but we blend them as we go. This makes them hard to notice, even for those who go through them. At one moment we may slip out of one stage back to another. But when we grow in our relationship with God we live more and more in stages three and four, loving God for God's sake and loving self for God's sake.

Behind these four stages lies questions such as, "what is love?" and "why do we love?" and these can send us into a discussion from which there is no reasonable way to conclude what love is at all. How do we teach a visitor from another planet what love really is if he has never even heard of love? But we must pursue these love-relationship questions in some way if we are to discover the deepest level of love ourselves, because *love is freedom*. Somehow we sense that. We know that the most loving people are the most free, but how did they get there? The lines from the song, "Why do I love you? Why do you love me?" are a symbol of the enigma of love when we try to analyze it without feeling it.

I found it helpful to ask my son Trevor one night at bedtime, "Why do you love me, Trevor?" and without a moment of hesitation he said, "Because you love me." Simply put, love turns out to be a response to someone who has already felt something about us. When we were young we learned love from someone who loved us and then we learned how to pass it on as we grew. But the trouble with love is sometimes we fall in love with ourselves. That's where Bernard of Clairvaux's four stages can help. By looking at them we can more clearly see the steps to new freedom in our love relationship with God.

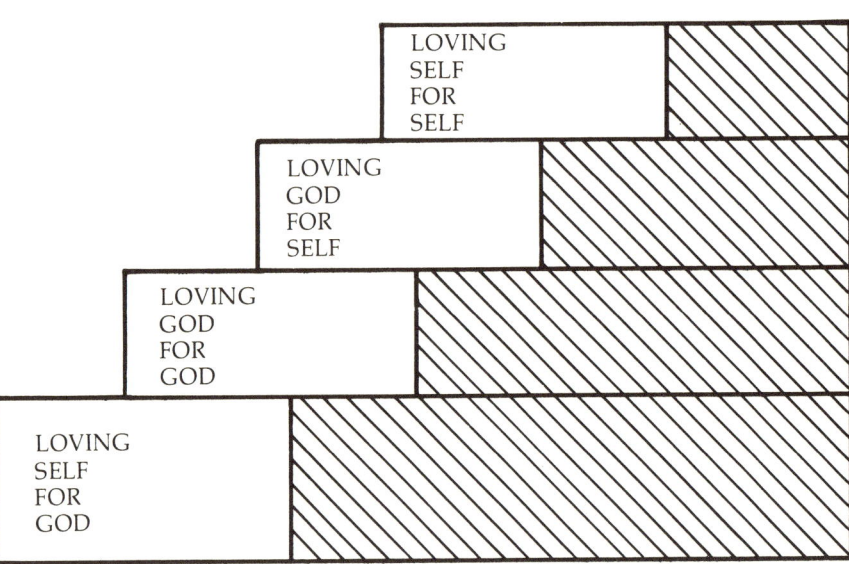

Step one, loving self for self's sake is a very honest step. If we pretend not to love self we are hypocrites. No person who ever lived got through life without caring about himself. No man ever hates his own flesh, according to the Apostle Paul. If we say that love is at least wishing good for someone we know we have loved ourselves, however selfless we may feel we are. So let's take a look at St. Bernard's first stage as honestly as we can.

Loving self for self's sake faces the fact that we are individuals. No carbon copies exist, as Bob Dresser put it in our breakfast meeting. This points to the Creator. We are the highest form of God's creation in this world. We were made with the capacity to be lovely. But the fact is we are often unlovely. That's where sin comes in.

Our Judaeo-Christian belief tells us sin is a defect. It's an addition caused by Satan, rather than the core of man and woman as created by God. So, not to love self is to despise Gods' handiwork. Since we are made in the image of God for fellowship with God we are to appreciate what he has created and be thankful.

But this notion of loving self for self can move away from honest gratitude to God toward indulgence of ourselves. That is the bad side of step one. While self-acceptance is a sign of our gratitude, self-preoccupation is a sign of indulgence. We are to care for God's handiwork but we are not to worship anything God has produced, and that includes ourselves.

The next stage, loving God for self's sake, becomes evident in our prayers of petition. Jesus said, "Ask and it shall be given you." There is nothing wrong in asking. We show God by our actions that we trust him when we ask him to help us. This, too, is an honest thing because we are admitting that we need help. This second stage is an infant stage in the sense that it is a pure learning time. It is both a level of need and response that is warm and loving. Here, we are invited to God's come-as-you-are-party and we are given nourishment. In true infancy this stage looks something like this.

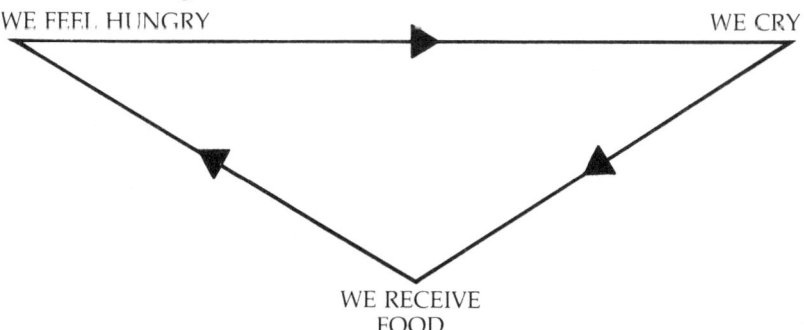

WE FEEL HUNGRY   WE CRY

WE RECEIVE
FOOD

This is a self-repeating, central feeling we grow up with. "If we trust God," we say to ourselves in our reflective moods, "we will receive something we need." The Christian life is intended to be a life of trusting a nourishing God and thanking him for the nurture we receive. All of us go through this stage in our physical and spiritual lives, and we return to it whenever we have real needs. It is a good stage because we relearn how to be dependent. "Suffer the little children to come to me" is a message to all of us. We are to allow ourselves to come to Christ as often as we have needs—and we will always be needy children in a very real sense.

But there is a bad side of this stage, as well. It is the "give me" attitude that we sometimes fall into. It's the things stage. We can't stay in a me-centered stage like this forever and really be loving in a mature way. We are to learn how to return God's love by becoming a caring person, and that's where stage three comes in.

Loving God for God's sake is going beyond blessing to find communion with the blesser. Just being together with someone we love is enough. We don't need to do anything. When I first visited my son Kevin and his wife in their new appartment in Cheyenne, Wyoming, I found it very enjoyable just to be there. They wanted to show me their town and take me places that would show me they cared, but I didn't need that. "We don't need to go anywhere," I said. "I'm just enjoying being here." It was a time of quiet contemplation for me. I loved them not for what they would do for me but for just being themselves.

Loving God for God and not for what he gives us is a new kind of awareness. We understand this only when we begin to realize that through a member of God's family named Jesus we can just "be". To know Jesus is to watch him at work and to love him. We reach this level of love through thinking, appreciating prayer or "being" prayer. When we say, "I'm just happy to be here with you, Lord," we have come to a point of appreciating our Lord for what he is, not just for what he does. Adam's sin caused him not to want to just "be" but to "do." Although there is nothing wrong with empasizing doing something in life, there is something wrong with a life of achievement that overlooks the quality of our relationship. Adam and Eve traded relationship for independent achievement. One of the most profound realizations we come to in the middle of stressful living is that achievement without relationship is stressful in itself. That kind of lopsided living is very lonely.

Loving God for God's sake is the beginning of a deeper relationship. When we say, "I love you, Lord, whether you do anything for me or not," we are learning to love God in the way he has already loved us. He authored this kind of love without any conditions whatever, and he showed it when he commissioned Jesus to become a brother on earth. God knew the difference between accepting us and accepting our sin. He never has accepted sin, but he has already accepted us for what we are. Jesus showed this accepting kind of love for us just by coming and "being" with us. He knew this same kind of accepting love the night before he died, when he realized more deeply than ever that he wasn't going to get anything out of his life on earth except the opportunity to love us as God wanted us to be loved. In doing that he gave us a model of loving God for God's sake. We repeat that kind of love, even though in a lesser way, every time we enter into

step three. We don't discover it so much by forcing ourselves to enter this phase but by responding to God's love.
We reach a point of feeling that God has done so much for
us that we want to do something for him. Even the unpleasant things. "Just for you, Lord," we say when we
truly reach step three. If God were to ask us at this stage,
"Why do you love me?" we sould say without a second
thought, "Because you love me, Lord."

That's the way it worked with a young inventor I knew
several years ago whose ideas were recognized by the
United States Government and by at least one manufac-
turer. "I felt a desire to return something for what God
had allowed me to discover," he said. It worked something like that, too, with Walter Hoving, Chairman of the
Board of Tiffany & Company, the world-famous New
York jewelry store that has become an institution. "I
needed a million dollars at one point in my career," he told
me one day, sitting in his wood panelled office above Fifth
Avenue. "I didn't have the money and I was about to lose
an investment opportunity that I felt we should make.
Then, suddenly, the money was granted by some of the
people right in the room, during a recess in our negotia-
tions. That's what made me realize that I owed God something," he said. When I left Walter Hoving's office, he gave
me a silver pin that said, "Try God." It was one of the pins
that Tiffany and Company produces for the benefit of a
Christian home for girls and women in trouble. It seemed
to me that he had entered a stage beyond receiving God's
gifts to a stage of returning God's love. The pin didn't say
"Try God for self" it just said "Try God."

How do we return God's love? By responding to the
clear and simple statement of Jesus, "If you love me keep

my commandments." After a while, sometimes years after becoming a Christian, we realize that it is impossible to keep the commandments of Jesus without loving him—for his sake. Then we are able to see the beginning of God's wisdom and feel the desire to be released from a less mature love that depends only on receiving. At that point we get a vision of how separate we are from caring for God's kingdom, because we have been concerned about *our* kingdom. Then we reach the point of confession-prayer on a new level. There is freedom in growing into this level.

But we still have not reached the point of loving self for God's sake. Bernard of Clairvaux's fourth phase of relationship is a new level of freedom—from anger as much as anything. The reason we cannot accept ourselves as God accepts us is that there is a gap between our behavior and our notions of what we ought to be. Impatience with ourselves reveals our high opinion of what we want to believe we are and our fleeting realization that we are not what we want to be. If God loves us unconditionally, even though he doesn't always like what we do, then why can't we love ourselves unconditionally, even though *we* might not like what we do?

We can blow the whole relationship with God out the window either by falling in love with ourselves or by hating ourselves. Either way we are preoccupied with us when we could be preoccupied with God. We could spend the rest of our lives atoning for our shortcomings and beating ourselves on the chest and miss the opportunity to accept ourselves for what we are. When we accept ourselves we can move on. We can't love God with all our heart and soul and mind if we are too busy thinking about our imperfections. We are to accept ourselves with our imperfections because God accepts us that way. While we are yet sinners (imperfect) we are to move on to the more important place of letting God do the changing in us, just by confessing our sins and repenting of them. We can move out of a life of feeling sorry or angry or of feeling anything that is mostly "me-thinking."

We can move out of worrying about judgments of our behavior in the eyes of someone else and even our own judgment of ourselves! We can stop living for the approval of people, no matter who they are. Moving out of ego preoccupation, whether it comes from achievement-oriented success or depression over lack of achievement, allows us to move into real commitment to the God who knows what needs changing in us and knows how to do it. By accepting ourselves—not trying to perfect ourselves—and letting Christ atone for us, we don't need to be lost in our own analysis paralysis.

The beauty of working in God's kingdom is that we never work alone. Relationship with God leads us to relationship with others. Loving God for God's sake and self for God's sake makes us love others for God's sake. Now, at this stage, we really have time for loving someone else.

Listen to what happened to a mother in her thirties. She had developed a heart flutter that the doctors couldn't explain or cure. She came to see Joan and me, and we asked her why she didn't like herself. It seemed clear that she was beating herself emotionally. While we talked, Joan and I prayed for wisdom. We didn't do it aloud, nor did we know until later what each other's prayers were. During our discussion our young visitor discovered that she didn't like her mother because of some things her mother had done years before. She wanted to like her but couldn't. She discovered that she didn't even like herself because she couldn't like her mother. An old hurt had been buried down so deep that it was literally giving her heart failure. Further, her father died when she was young and she had never forgiven God for taking her father away. Once she saw what had happened there was no need to go any further with the cause of her stressful condition.

We searched together for God's cure as we talked. "For some reason that we all find hard to understand," we said to her, "God requires us to forgive others before we can be forgiven ourselves. What you need to do is forgive your mother so you can understand what forgiveness is. Then God will forgive you and you will be able to forgive yourself." The impact of God's plan of forgiveness rushed in on her suddenly as we sat talking with her. She prayed with the tearful, chestful sobs of a person who had been carrying a heavy weight of anger around for years. "Lord," she prayed, still crying softly, "I forgive my mother." Then after some tears of relief she prayed, "I forgive you for taking my father, Lord. Please forgive me, too." She was forgiven while we sat nearby, and we never heard her complain of heart trouble after that. Her heart trouble was spiritual first, then physical, but both heart conditions were healed in one night!

So often we struggle with ourselves, knowing we shouldn't dislike ourselves, yet not knowing why we do. We need to see the difference between liking *imperfections in* oneself and loving oneself—and we need to know deep down inside the freeing power of forgiveness. The words,

"Let not your heart be troubled," are words for us today. So are the words in The Lord's Prayer, ". . . Forgive us our trespasses as we forgive those who trespass against us." These heartfelt words can free us from the deeper stress that can beset us for years.

The steps or stages of love we have been considering are ways to respond to Christs' commandment that we are to love God with all our heart and soul and mind. But Jesus adds a second commandment before we really have time to absorb the first one. He leaps right into the neighbor issue. Forgiveness heals neighbors. Forgiveness is an absolute necessity to love. We can't love self for self, God for self, God for God, or self for God without forgiveness. New freedom to love God and our neighbors with all our heart requires us to remove anything that is occupying our heart already. Forgiveness empties our hearts of the things that block love. We simply can't be heart-free without it. When we forgive we can be forgiven. We are promised that by God who has been ready to forgive all along. But there is one final requirement that God makes before we can have deep freedom. Christ said, "If your brother has something against you, go and make it right and then come back to my altar," (*Matthew 5:23,24* author's paraphrase). That seems so unfair at first, until we realize that a brother who feels hurt may have been hurt because of something we have done and didn't know about. Even if we have done nothing wrong and a brother thinks we have, *we* become free when we go and set it right. If someone is hurting because of our actions and we don't want to go to him, we may have a dark corner in our heart.

A new and deeper freedom comes to those who have no

dark corners. Then enthusiasm comes. Not pasted-on or worked-up enthusiasm, but deep down enthusiasm. Now we are ready to discover what enthusiasm really is. That is vital if we are going to be free of stressful living. But we need a simple way to *keep* enthusiasm at work in our lives. How we go about doing that is answered in the next chapter, "How to Get Real Enthusiasm."

Fifteen

How to Get
Real Enthusiasm

There are at least two reasons why everybody likes enthusiasm. Real enthusiasm not only excites us, it is good for
us as well.

Enthusiasm can be as contagious in a good way as
catching a cold is in a harmful way. When we catch enthusiasm the dis-ease of our stress is forgotten for a time,
because real enthusiasm is the answer to stressful living.
But what is "real" enthusiasm?

Real enthusiasm isn't a particular kind of feeling. Sometimes enthusiasm bubbles up and overflows. At other
times it is a deep well of feeling within that quietly re-
freshes and strengthens us in the depths of sorrow. Whatever the feeling, there is one thing certain about enthusiasm: When we find it it is always *in* someone, never in
things, and that's what makes it look different at different
times in different people.

Take a look at an evangelical church in the middle of a
joyful hymn-sing. We can hear the words, "I've got the
joy, joy, joy, joy down in my heart." There's no question
that excitement abounds, and it builds with each song.
"I'm inright, outright, upright, downright happy all the
time," sings the entire congregation of happy people. By

this time the church is filled with excitement, but that may
or may not be real enthusiasm.

Imagine we have just dropped in to see the spiritual
musical, "Your Arm's Too Short to Box with God." It
radiated excitement since the opening on Broadway.
When we take our seat we realize we are in a packed
theater with an all-black cast and a 90 percent black audience. The performance takes off like a rocket. Halfway
through a pulsating musical number a performer with
dynamic charisma looks out at the audience and asks, "Do
you feel the power?" All around us the answer is "yes."
"But do you *feel* the power?" he asks. "Yes," says the
crowd, clapping their hands. "Have you *got* the power?"
"Yes," says a beaming person right next to us, and suddenly we wish we had been able to say it, too. "Do you
want the power?" asks the man on stage. "Yes," roars the
crowd and some of them are standing up, to our surprise.
Now a 300-pound woman sitting in the next seat has
really caught the feeling, and we can't help but catch it as
her seat rocks back and 300 pounds of excitement suddenly stand up, dragging us up with her. When that much
excitement stands up we've got to go with it or be buried
by it. It either ignites us or scares us to death, and we
really feel it. But even that may not be real enthusiasm.

The real thing comes in all kinds of packages and in all
kinds of ways. We can live right next to someone with
enthusiasm and not catch it, or we can catch it when no
one seems around—perhaps while looking at a sunlit
stream rippled by a soft breeze—when we suddenly feel
the Spirit of the Lord saying, "I made this for you and me
to enjoy today." Enthusiasm is the spirit of life *within* the
world we see and feel. The word enthusiasm, literally

drawn from the words "en" and "theos" or "God within," isn't trumped up, pasted on or injected into our bodies. It comes to us when we let go of our isolated search for happiness or peace or excitement and invite in the source of enthusiasm.

Let's go all the way back to the incident where the woman from Sychar was offered real enthusiasm while looking for a bucket of water. Then we will look at a day-by-day way to obtain enthusiasm for ourselves.

"Jesus was tired from the long walk in the hot sun and sat wearily beside the well (outside Sychar). Soon a Samaritan woman came to draw water, and Jesus asked her for a drink. He was alone at the time as his disciples had gone into the village to buy some food. The woman was surprised that a Jew would ask a 'despised Samaritan' for anything—usually they wouldn't even speak to them!—and she remarked about this to Jesus.

"He replied, 'If you only knew what a wonderful gift God has for you, and who I am, you would ask me for some *living* water!'

"'But you don't have a rope or a bucket,' she said, 'And this is a very deep well! Where would you get this living water? And besides, are you greater than our ancestor Jacob? How can you offer better water than this which he and his sons and cattle enjoyed?'

"Jesus replied that people soon become thirsty again after drinking this water. 'But the water I give them,' he said, 'becomes a perpetual spring within them, watering them forever with eternal life.'

"'Please, sir," the woman said, "give me some of that water! Then I'll never be thirsty again and won't have to make this long trip out here every day.'"

This incident from the fourth chapter of John in the Living Bible shows our human desire for new life on our own terms. It is like that today in our search for release from stress. We want a once-and-for-all drink of water so we can be complete in ourselves—so we won't have to go out of our own way to get some more water. But that's not the way enthusiasm works. Enthusiasm is a dependent relationship. It's on-going. It is day-by-day worship that we never outgrow. People who live stressful lives are always trying to grow out of dependence in order to be complete in themselves. But the answer to stressful living is to learn how to let real enthusiasm spring up in us, and that happens in a daily practice of dependent worship, rather than adoration-worship or fear-worship that we might have in a visit to a cathedral or church.

". . . It's not *where* we worship that counts," Jesus said, "but *how* we worship—is our worship spiritual and real? Do we have the Holy Spirit's help? For God is Spirit, and we must have his help to worship as we should. The Father wants this kind of worship from us" (John 4:21-24 LB).

This kind of dependent worship overcomes stressful living. Yet when we look around at our neighbors, including some who are committed Christians, we find they certainly are not stress-free. And we know that we are not totally stress-free ourselves, even after several years of living in the Christian way. Certainly our nation is not stress-free. Even Christ experienced stress, although he was not guilty of stressful living. Yet we are guilty of stressful living a good share of our Christian lives. That's because we haven't yet learned to be dependent.

Have you ever heard someone say, "I believe God

wants me to make my own decisions. Once I have given him my life I believe he trusts me to live as I should." This license to live separate from God is another one of life's big lies that keeps many otherwise committed people from finding full enthusiasm and freedom from stressful living. That kind of thinking happens to all of us, but it seems especially believable to the rational people who are used to planning their lives in intimate detail. People who have had success in the details of their lives find it especially difficult to really worship God dependently, day by day. You can almost see them saying by their actions, "Now that I've become a Christian how can *I* work things out so I will live successfully?" Sometimes that mental set doesn't happen right away. It can happen to us after being a Christian for years. It's when independence becomes a pattern of life that the dryness of stressful living sets in again. The reason is we don't let the water of real enthusiasm flow in the intimate, moment-by-moment details of our lives. We become "dry Christians," who forget to drop the bucket down into the perpetual spring within us. After a while we become as wells without water, in effect, even though the water of Christ's Spirit is available down deep.

For the Christian there really is no such thing as the word "I." It's we or it's nothing at all. One of my sons sat with me one evening talking about the many thoughts he had been going through about marriage. "Sometimes I think I know what I should do in selecting a wife, dad. But at other times I am lost." We talked for hours and finally came to the conclusion that we couldn't figure out wife selection. "I don't think you're supposed to try, son," I said. "Marrying the right partner is something God is better able to decide for you. At least you don't have to make the decision alone. Sometimes it's awfully stressful even to try. But there is a way to get the right answer without so much worry."

My son was trying to come to a logical conclusion about something that there is no logical conclusion for. We began to see once again that we aren't supposed to figure out everything in life. That kind of total independence just isn't available to us. We are to be enthused by being dependent when we approach any life decision such as marriage or a new job or the right school to attend. When my son and I prayed at midnight, I heard him say, "Forgive me, Lord, for the worry I have been allowing. Show me your way in this." I saw the release in him then. "That's good, dad," he said.

Here's how we can tap God's perpetual spring today and renew a life of stress-releasing enthusiasm.

1. When you are anxious about or troubled by some circumstance or relationship confess the sin of living or acting independently from God. Tell him today—this moment—that you are moving over and letting him flow into your day and into yourself.

2. Commit yourself to his way again by asking, "What shall I do today, Lord, with this particular problem?"

3. Then simply do what seems right to do, regardless of how little or out of sequence or ill-timed it may appear to be. That is dependent worship. That is also how to get real enthusiasm.

Dependent worship really works in stressful lives. It's exactly the kind of worship Jesus was talking about.

What would happen if the entire country started living in dependent worship like this? What if every day we were to start out with the question, "What shall I do today, Lord?" Let's take a look, not only at what would happen, but at what has happened when this question is used in the three steps to enthusiasm just outlined.

I was manager of three secretaries as a part of my duties in running a department. We were conducting management development schools for a major division of my corporation at a conference center owned by a separate company. In order to be close to our schools we leased what space we could at the conference center, but the space for the secretaries was cramped. They kept getting in one another's way. It was like having three cooks in one little kitchen, and it wasn't working at all. It was the story of territorial rights that gets nations into trouble, only this time it was three secretaries in trouble. Each one had real strengths but was crowded by the fear of her talents being cramped.

I knew I was doing a bad job with the problem because I was spending my time doing the things I wanted to do—teaching, speaking, writing—everything but managing the problem. Finally, when I was forced by the unhappiness of the three secretaries to deal with their concerns I saw how big the task was and how insufficient I was to handle it, in spite of my management experience. I asked the secretaries for their day-to-day work preferences and then for a list of the things they had to do but didn't like to to. I told them that I would spread the enjoyable work assignments among them—as well as the undesirable work. When I had talked to each one separately and received her preferences I was faced with the Solomon-like task of making three people happy, not just two. How do you slice the good work three ways?

Late at night when all my family was asleep, I stared at the preferences of the three secretaries and my scribbled plans to re-arrange the work assignments. I knew that a physical move and more space would help, but I saw, too, that wherever we were our three secretaries must always work with team spirit if we were to get our job done. I faced the truth then that I really had to care about *their* interests at work, not just my own work interests. At midnight I asked, "What shall I do, Lord? I need your wisdom in this." Then I just wrote down what seemed right and discussed it the next day with my management colleagues. When we agreed, I called the secretaries together and showed what we would do. All three came away from our meeting with a real willingness to start over. It wasn't what I said, alone, or the changes I had come up with. It was relinquishing what I wanted to do and inviting God to show me what he wanted to do, and that was to begin to change our hearts. But we had to keep working at the changes in our work circumstances and relationships on a day-to-day basis. One burst of insight alone doesn't always change our day-to-day practice. It just changes our willingness to come to the problem differently.

"What shall I do today, Lord?" is a question that becomes more powerful as we use it everyday. It becomes a practical way to live *in* enthusiasm. When we ask the question any time we are perplexed or troubled by today's circumstances or relationships we begin to abandon our own way and be healed of it through day-by-day practice.

Look one more time at Hebrews 4, verses 7 through 11, this time at J. B. Phillips' translation. This famous "rest" chapter includes the ancient words of King David when he talked about the children of Israel losing their dependence in the wilderness. "Today if ye shall hear his voice, harden not your hearts. For if Joshua had given them the rest, (a long time ago, in the wilderness) we should not find God saying, at a much later date, 'today.' There still exists, therefore, a full and complete rest for the people of God. And he who experiences his rest is resting from his own work as fully as God from his."

King David's words apply to people in our day. This *today* kind of dependency is really the kind of obedient living that God has been pointing us toward all along. We don't understand the kind of release that comes from it until we try it. No amount of talking or reading about this kind of enthusiasm is of any use until we try it, today—with our real concerns. Then the question becomes even more timely. "What shall I do now, Lord?" And that becomes a moment-by-moment kind of living that helps in the four circumstances and four relationships we looked at earlier in depth.

When we look at relationships with our spouse, children, parents and self in an obedient and confident spirit we are more ready to be healed of *our* way of dealing with our relationships. When we look at vexing circumstances such as financial, health, career, and time pressures in the spirit of "What shall I do now, Lord?" we are more ready to be healed of our tendency to be overcome by yesterday's problems. The dis-ease of stressful living is "piled-up living." It is a life of carry-over from yesterday's unresolved relationships and circumstances.

What is our real problem? It's whatever we haven't really dealt with that continues to trouble us, perhaps because we are afraid to really see ourselves as we are or to trust God to guide us, because he might want to lead in a different way from our own way. But if our way hasn't worked for the past several days or months or years we need to break out of the prison of our set ways, and into the freedom that is his. We work our way out day-by-day before we learn how to be free moment-by-moment.

One of the besetting problems we all face is time pressure and how to deal with it. When my manager, Ed Kappus, and I spent a day at the office looking at our work responsibilities and goals we stumbled onto an idea that has really helped us in our time management. We made a pact that we would be willing to let our weaknesses be known to each other in order to deal more throughly with them. It was a spontaneous kind of decision that just came to us as we discussed our individual time management needs and our work responsibilities. Out of that relationship we began to step into a whole new territory of the freedom to be weak, rather than the human tendency to allow only our strengths to be seen on the job.

That relationship was a frightening one at times but a healing one, too. Out of it I began to see that I must do the important but unpleasant things in life, as well as the enjoyable ones. But then I found that the urgent and the pleasant things in life kept crowding out the important but unpleasant things, and I knew I needed help. That's where the question at the beginning of the day, "What shall I do today, Lord?" began to free me to do the important things moment-by-moment. I began to realize that God knows what is important and he is interested in the intimate details of what I do, because what I do is important to him. By first asking him what I should do I began to get the perspective I needed, and toward the end of the year I found that I was actually living in new territory. By December 31st I had done virtually everything I was supposed to do and I had begun to live more free from the guilt of unfinished responsibilities.

When we ask God, "what shall I do today?" he puts his hand on whatever needs doing in his kingdom, even beyond our own lives. At Christmas time Kevin and Diane brought our brand new granddaughter home to see us. It was our first look at Kimberley. When the three of them emerged from the exit ramp at Kennedy Airport, Kimberley was as quiet as a little doll. Her big brown eyes were rolling around just looking at everything, and I fell in love with her right away. Kimberley was to be christened during their visit, and we found ourselves a few days later in a little Catholic church in upstate New York, looking on as the priest went through the ceremony. It was all so strange to our Protestant ears. We felt the words had just been tumbled out without feeling. There was only a handful of us there, trying to follow along as the priest paused for the briefest of instants to say, "page 10" and race on again, speaking what looked like such important words, if we could catch up. I could feel the anger rising in me at the machine-gun rapidity of the ceremony. Perhaps I was angry at the fact that my own father had not been invited. I knew he would have been a warm and personal part of the ceremony. Suddenly the ceremony was over, and I had not seen a sign that anyone cared, except that the priest left with the mumbled words, "Drive safely, now."

I carried my anger around for two days until I really

could ask God for help in order to forgive the priest. "Help me to forgive him, Lord," I prayed and then the question came to me. "What shall I do now, Lord?" I began to see that I was all wrapped up in my hurt feelings when the priest may have been a needy person, too. Why would he rattle through such a sacred event? I remembered then the comment from one of the parishioners of the little Catholic church. "Don't you just love our priest? He can say the mass so fast we can be home in half an hour." I realized that the priest may have fallen into the trap of ladling out fast ceremonies because that was all the parish wanted. Had anyone ever gone to the priest and said, "I care?" Had anyone thought for years that the priest was a neighbor, a real person who lived alone in a rambling rectory and came and went with just a nod and a hurried smile from his parishioners? I realized then that he would never be able to look at his own Kimberley and know what it is to see his granddaughter dressed all in white, looking around with big brown trusting eyes. When I thought of these things I began to consider the priest.

When we ask the question "What shall I do now, Lord?" we open ourselves to God's perspective, not ours, and enthusiasm begins in the middle of hurt. I talked of my feelings with a group of men that I meet and pray with weekly. Charlie, an Episcopal priest in the group was especially helpful to me. "I would be angry too," he said. "But God may have something in store for the priest out of this."

"I've been thinking of writing him a letter," I said. But my group said, "No. Call him." Then I realized I should not only call him but ask to see him. Strangely, I began to care very much for the priest. A few days later I was traveling through the little town, and I called the priest to see if I could talk with him. "You may," he said. "I'll leave the front door open."

I stopped at my sister-in law's house to leave my eleven-year-old son Trevor there before visiting the priest. Trevor's words seemed filled with God's wisdom as we parted. "Don't be too hard on him, dad," he said, "and may the Lord be in your words."

Knowing that I was on a trip that God wanted to direct I asked my sister-in-law Barbara to pray with me just before going.

When I arrived at the old rectory I had not prepared any particular thing to say because I wanted to be open to what God wanted me to do next.

"Mr. Osgood," the priest said, "tell me what troubled you about the ceremony."

"I was angry at you." I said, "But I'm not angry with you now." Not knowing what to do next I said, "I'm coming to you as a brother in Christ because I told others in the parish I was angry, but I didn't tell you."

"I'm grateful that you came. You don't know how grateful," he said, looking at me earnestly.

"I just thought by coming I would be helped and perhaps you would be too."

"Yes," he said, looking at me in a very open way.

From then on I was not aware of any awkwardness because God seemed very much in control of our talk. The priest who had seemed so careless was so humble and loving now that I was struck with the spirit of brotherhood about him. It seemed right to ask if we could pray together, then.

"You lead, Mr. Osgood," he said. But the real message for me was when he prayed, because he asked for forgiveness in such a spirit of humility. He prayed for his parish and reflected on the sufferings of Jesus with such sweetness that I couldn't keep back the quiet tears. And I suddenly loved him very much.

Still not knowing what to say when our prayers were over I asked, "Is the Lord Jesus in your heart?" It could have been such a presumptuous, probing question of a priest, but it wasn't that at all. It was just a time for affirming something very important to both of us. "You'd better believe it," he said with tenderness. "I spend time with Jesus early every morning. When the doorbell or the phone rings my prayer is, "Jesus, be with me." We parted with a bear hug then—a manly and emotional one.

Out in the car again I was awed with the power of God to heal when we open ourselves to his indwelling presence. A deeper enthusiasm had returned out of my hurt.

The way to live free of ourselves is by the enthusiasm of God's Spirit, according to J. B. Phillips in his translation of Galatians 5:16 through 26. "Here is my advice," says Paul, "Live your whole life in the Spirit and you will not satisfy the desires of your lower nature. For the whole energy of the lower nature is set against the Spirit, while the whole power of the Spirit is contrary to the lower nature. Here is the conflict and that is why you are not free to do what you want to do. But if you follow the leading of the Spirit, you stand clear of the law."

"The activities of the lower nature are obvious. Here is a list: sexual immorality, impurity of mind, sensuality, worship of false gods, witchcraft, hatred, quarreling, jealousy, bad temper, rivalry, factious, party-spirit, envy, drunkenness, orgies and things like that. I solemnly assure you, as I did before, that those who indulge in such things will never inherit God's kingdom. The Spirit, however, produces in human life fruits such as these: love, joy, peace, patience, kindness, generosity, fidelity, tolerance and self-control—and no law exists against any of them.

"Those who belong to Christ Jesus have crucified their old nature with all that it loved and lusted for. If our lives are centered in the Spirit, let us be guided by the Spirit. Let us not be ambitious for our own reputations, for that only means making each other jealous." Those words of advice mean more to us as we live them daily—and as we grow into moment-by-moment freedom.

We are standing, now, you and I, at the threshold of a bold new frontier of living. There is a promised land that we can occupy just as our ancient cousins, the children of Israel, were told they could occupy. They didn't go in, but we can. Freedom from the dis-ease of stressful living is just across the border of our willingness to be changed. We won't find complete freedom from stress when we cross the border, because change itself is stressful. But we will find freedom from our *lifestyle* of living. We can use any of the hints for release we have considered in the chapters of this book, but the real answer is in a day-by-day dependent relationship with God who wants to enthuse us. By plunging into his kingdom and watching him unfold his plan we learn how to love him with our heart and soul and mind, and to love our neighbor as ourself. There is tearful, joyful peace in his way to our own promised land. But we now know that the journey is accomplished a step at a time, and that there are many refreshing wells of water along the way when we drop our bucket down deep by asking, "What shall I do *now*, Lord?" That is the question we must ask with all our heart to live free of our stressful lives. And the promise is freedom now, not freedom for tomorrow. Freedom comes in the very moment we believe that our Lord *is now* answering our questions. We don't even need to know what he wants us to do. As we trust him, moment by moment, we *are free*! This freedom brings us to a place where we can truly understand the Christian's response to stress.

Sixteen

What Is the Christian's Response to Stress?

When I told a colleague the subtitle of this book he said, "Is there a difference in the way a Christian handles stress?" I said, "Yes, there is." After reading about the pressure points that we all face and relating to them as a Christian throughout this book, we now know there is a difference, but what is it exactly?

If we agree that stress really is within us and that it is caused by any number of pressure points that make us uncomfortable, to say the least, and even desperate at times, then we begin to see that it is our *response* to stress that makes the difference, not the pressure itself. That is the key to stress management. It isn't what goes into a person or what touches his life that is so important. It's what comes from a person. That idea, expressed by Jesus in another context, applies specifically to stress as well.

Throughout the chapters of this book we have been considering specific causes of stress and reflecting on our own internal response, whether or not we have been calling ourselves Christians. But the responses presented in the preceding chapters have been intended to show how a Christian *does* respond as opposed to how he *can* respond to stress. Your life and mine are examples of imperfect dealings with stress when we try to respond to it without help. Christ is telling us to live with stress, but never to live with it alone. Relationship is the key. Not with just anyone, as helpful as that can be, but with him. Literally, any cause of stress is faced easier that way. The pressure point isn't changed, but *we are changed*. We are literally enabled to handle pressure better from within.

Let's look at the Christians in the Book of Acts. When you put this book down I hope the next book you pick up will be the Acts of the Apostles, because it shows what *came out* of some Christians who were living in acutely stressful times. They experienced many pressure points, but they were full of joy at being considered worthy to experience them. Remember when they were thrown in prison just for telling about Christ? Remember when they were beaten, even before being tried, and warned not to talk about Jesus? Steven was killed for doing just that. The reason he could handle that experience and even say, "Forgive them, Lord . . . ," was that he was doing what God wanted him to do, from the inside out.

All of that sounds so idealistic and perhaps even impossible today. But we can have the living-with-Christ experience only by inviting Christ into whatever relationship or circumstances we have at this moment, so he can live it with us. What will come out of us is what is in us—*his* response.

The Christian response to stress is not to have a goal to be happy. It is not to try to avoid stress. That will come anyway. To spend our lives trying to avoid stress is to find it sneaking in the back door. The Christian response is to accept the stress that comes and respond to it—not as Christ would if he were here but as Christ within us responds for us. To try by ourselves to live up to the way Christ did respond is itself stressful. But to literally get out of the way and let Christ respond in us and through us is to deal with it in the most effective way ever known. The remarkable discovery we make as we reread the Book of Acts is that they were never alone.

While reflecting on this book during the closing days of a hectic personal schedule, I realized that one more chapter was needed, but that I had run out of time. We were already beyond the date for the manuscript to be at the printer. In discussing this with my editor at Christian Herald, and in my mad dash for another airplane moments later, I realized that I would not be able to get the chapter done alone. In an overnight trip to Atlanta, I was to be reminded that I am never alone in the middle of any pressure point.

I caught the plane with minutes to spare and began writing on the way. In the hotel in Atlanta I continued to write. The words that came out had to do with getting God's rest—a similar message to the first chapter of this book, where we considered the importance God placed on resting from his own work on the seventh day. But this was not to be the real message.

The next morning while in the shower I realized that the Christian response to stress is not rest alone. We weren't created to rest. That was just *one* of the things God wanted us to remember. The deeper message was still something more. When I appeared in the hotel lecture room, I began to experience the deeper message so subtly that I didn't recognize it for hours. It was after three events that I began to understand it.

The first incident occurred when the person who introduced me before I gave a management lecture found out that I was a Christian. He said, "I am, too." Then he said quietly when I left, "God bless you." That wasn't profound because it had happened before.

The second experience occurred on the way to the airport in the cab when an African-American driver overheard my comment to another person in the cab that I was trying to complete the final chapter of a book on the Christian's response to stress. He said, "Are you a Bible-believing Christian?" I said, "A born-again Bible-believing Christian." He grinned in the mirror and said, "I am, too." And he said, "Christians have an answer to stress because of the Spirit inside them."

The third experience happened on the plane to New York's LaGuardia Airport. I had arrived at the Atlanta airport check-in desk at 4:20 with a reservation for the 6:08. But a plane due to leave at 4:20 was late and there were a few seats left. I caught the 4:20 and was given a seat assignment beside a young woman. Within minutes she had said to me (I don't remember why), "Are you a Christian?" I said, "Yes," and she said, "I am, too." We talked about stress and my final chapter and she prayed while I wrote. One of the things she said was, "Good things always cost something." It was her way of commenting on stress in her own life. But that wasn't the whole message.

What each person said wasn't the new insight. It was the fact that three people were just there, *being* a message to me, while I was wrestling with the subject of the Christian's response to stress. A white man had gripped my hand, a black man had driven me to the airport, and a young woman had flown with me back to New York, and each had shown me what Christ wanted me to know deep down inside. He gives each of us the same message, just as he gave it to the Apostles and to people down through the years. To you at this moment as you read these final words about the Christian's response to stress, God is whispering, "You are not alone. You never were. I am waiting for you."

What is the Christian's response to stress? It is knowing that we never need to be lonely, and living in this knowledge in very practical ways. He is here in the middle of all our pressure points. The secret is in the prayer of Jesus when He knew He was going to die in a few days. It's found in the 17th chapter of John's Gospel, verse 20 through 26. Jesus could have asked the Heavenly Father to forget the experiment with people on earth. He could have said, "I guess we'll just need to wipe them out." Or he could have said, "Let's just re-program their minds." But what He prayed, in effect, was, "I want them to live *in* Me in the same way I live *in* You and You (the Father) live *in* Me. And I want this for all who ever believe." You and I can live in God, and we can be lived in. We can enjoy the greatest invitation of all time. Accepting the Great Invitation is the key. In His Spirit we live in freedom so real that we cannot describe it.

FOR FURTHER READING

Osgood, Don. *Listening for God's Silent Language.* Stamford, CT: Hitchhiker Books, 2000

Osgood, Don. *Fatherbond.* Stamford, CT: Hitchhiker Books, 2001 ed.

Osgood, Don. *How to Really Love Your Job.* Hitchhiker Books, 2002 ed.

Appendix

Are You Type A, B, or C?

Appendix: Are You Type A, B, or C?

Some years ago two doctors discovered that our personality type affects our reaction to stress. They said we tend to be either a Type A or a Type B person. When we read their reports about stressful Type A behavior we learn that it will have an affect on our hearts. When we consider the more relaxed Type B behavior we sense this will help us live a longer, happier life but our work life may suffer. But are we either A or B or nothing?

TYPE A

Type A people spend their lives rushing to meet schedules and accomplish things, almost as though they had to. Type B people seem less driven to achieve, sometimes not even thinking about getting something done. But there is a third type of behavior. We'll call it Type C because it is in a different dimension from A or B. Actually, these three behaviors, A, B and C, are at work in our everyday lives in varying styles or combinations. We'll explore some of these and the contributions of three authorities whose life work has an impact on our knowledge of stressful living: Dr. Hans Selye, a Canadian biological scientist; Dr. Abraham Maslow, an American behavioral humanist; and Jesus Christ. But first let's try to better understand Type A and B.

Dr. Meyer Friedman, of Mount Zion Hospital in San Francisco, has studied 3,000 people over the past 15 years to determine what causes heart failure. He has concluded that most people who are prone to heart failure fall into an A pattern of living. The common traits are excessive ambition, overwhelming aggression, marked impatience, and an obsession with time. In his opinion, these people, because of their driven or harassed lifestyle, suffer two-and-a-half times as many heart attacks as people who are called Type B. The Type A person may take up physical exercise to balance his life but even the exercise itself will be the competitive kind, whether it is a workout, tennis or jogging. In jogging, for example, the race is with the clock. How a person uses time is one clue. Type A walks fast, talks fast, drives hard and rushes headlong into anything and everything he or she takes on. Personal gain is the name of the game, and the true Type A never stops playing it. There is likely an underlying reason why this type has such drive. But whatever the reason, this person lives a life of dis-ease with the world and with self. He is out to prove or realize something, and is in a hurry to do it.

TYPE B

The more relaxed, easygoing Type B people are more accepting of life circumstances. They like to eat slowly and enjoy their meals, for instance. And when they participate in sports they play for fun as much as competition. Not all B's are out of the running as far as their careers are concerned. They have just learned a different approach. Some know how to be successful and happy, too. While the hard-driving A type may get more done in the short range, Type B has a better chance to live longer, and perhaps even achieve more in the long run. Without particularly thinking about it, Type B people ultimately can become A people, as well as the other way around. Even though a learned pattern generally sticks with a person after a few years and we tend to stay in our type, B people can be remade into A's through career or home pressures. Many people in sales were at one time really B people but they put on the A approach when they saw it as the way to conquer the sales territory. But our new patterns don't happen right away. An A person doesn't become a B overnight. If there is any change at all it is more likely a curing or maturing process than a cold-turkey approach.

An A person has an unsatisfied question about himself that drives him to find out his true worth. "A" people are intent on finding "how good can I get to be some day?" and never quite find out who they are today. At least they are never *really* satisfied.

Dr. Abraham Maslow had much to say about this drive for something better in several books and many articles in which he defined a set of unsatisfied needs that people go through in life. The first edition of his book, *Toward a Psychology of Being*, sold more than 100,000 copies. His position as chairman of the Department of Psychology at Brandeis University and earlier involvement as a teacher at Brooklyn College gave him a firm background in behavioral science. His service as president of the American Psychological Association in the late sixties indicated the place of respect he held in the psychological community. At times, he brought the theology of his Jewish heritage into his writings in an attempt to look closely at what makes people the way they are.

An easy way to think of Dr. Maslow's basic idea is to

think of people as having very specific and very strong needs that are satisfied as we go through life and make us want to satisfy the next level of needs. He says our basic needs are in a series of five steps. The first one is for the basic needs of life, such as food and shelter, the second is for safety and security, the third for belonging and affection, the fourth: respect and self-respect, and the fifth for self-actualization.

This ladder or pyramid of needs looks like this:

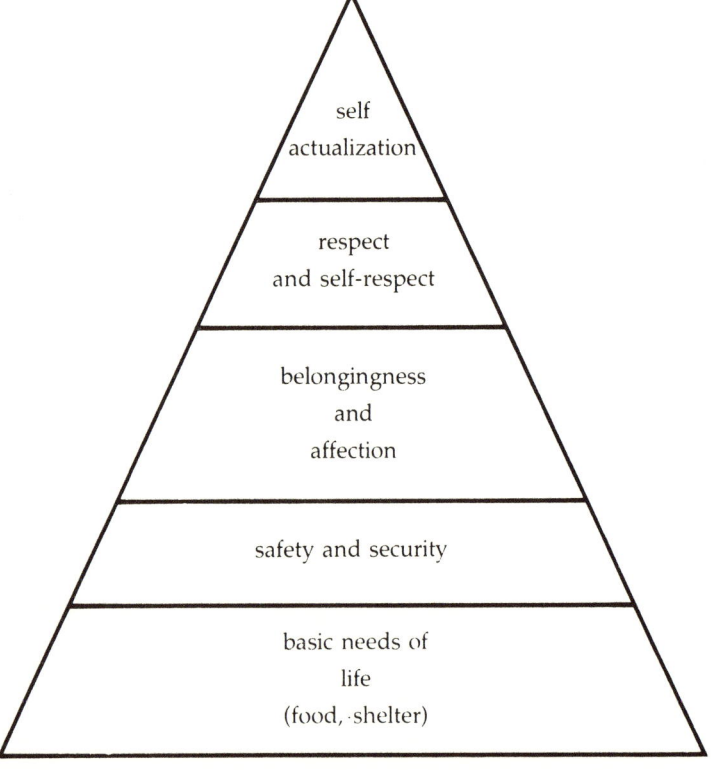

Abraham Maslow was so excited about the possibilities of his definition that he said in his book, *Toward a Psychology of Being*, "There is now emerging over the horizon a new conception of human sickness and of human health, a psychology that I find so thrilling and so full of wonderful possibilities that I yield to the temptation to present it publicly even before it is checked and confirmed, and before it can be called reliable scientific knowledge."

What Abraham Maslow wanted to do was present a "health psychology." If his assumptions were right he felt they would provide not only a scientific ethic but a natural value system, "a court of ultimate appeal for the determination of good and bad, of right and wrong."

"The more we learn about man's natural tendencies," he said, "the easier it will be to tell him how to be good, how to be happy, how to be fruitful, how to respect himself, how to love, how to fulfill his highest potentialities."

When Professor Maslow turned his attention to the person deep inside us, he talked about the "inner person" in a theological sense. "This inner nature," he said, "as much as we know of it so far, seems not to be intrinsically evil, but rather either neutral or positively 'good.'" If we study Maslow long enough we almost forget what Christ said about inner nature.

There are many others who have explored the inner nature of people from a psychological viewpoint. Among them are the famous behaviorists C. G. Jung, Carl Rogers, the American psychotherapist; and the Eastern Buddhists. Maslow's idea of the inner person is like theirs in many ways. All of them speak in one way or another about the attainment of the true self and the wholeness of personality. But all of them seem to have overlooked Christ's definition of the needs of the inner person, and of wholeness.

In the 1960's Dr. Hans Selye began to capture the attention of the medical world with his ideas about stress. As a biological scientist, Dr. Selye has been working on stress since 1936, and by the time he reached age 70, he had become known by many as "Dr. Stress." He was born in Vienna and followed a career as an endocrinologist before writing many of his 33 books and 1600 articles. His book *Stress without Distress* is printed in a number of languages. For years he was a faculty member of the University of Montreal before founding The International Institute of Stress. He says stress is a normal state of affairs and some is even pleasant. For instance, a person who gives a talk is under stress even while giving it successfully, but it is exciting and productive. This kind of healthy or productive stress he calls "eustress." The kind we think of, usually, is called "distress." In simple medical terms Dr. Selye defines stress as a nonspecific response of our body to any demand. He cites a number of ways that people can deal with stress, but added in an interview with *U.S. News and World Report*, "It cannot be handled easily. One person needs a clergyman, while another needs a psycho-analyst . . . Specialists have to be trained to deal with the stress of being a boss or an employee or a wife."

"Then there's really nowhere to turn for treatment at the present time?" asked an interviewer.

"Well, there are a few physicians specializing in stress diseases, but most of them are not very well trained. To tell you the truth, very few people know much about stress."

At the close of the interview Dr. Selye was asked, "If you had to give one piece of advice to people about stress, what would you say to them?"

"I would offer the wisdom of the Bible translated into terms a scientist can easily accept today: "Earn thy neighbor's love."

Listening to Dr. Selye's comments and thinking of Dr. Maslow we begin to realize that it's the attitude or the state of life we are in that is important. What we do with stress comes from this particular state.

Type A and B behavior as expressed by Drs. Friedman and Rosenman, the San Francisco heart specialists, are also states or attitudes of life. The reason these states are so intriguing to us is that they help answer a basic question that is stressful in itself, "Who Am I?"

In speaking to audiences across the United States for the American Management Association I see the same interest in finding answers to this and other simple but profound questions, such as "Where am I heading?" "How can I get where I want to go?" "Who is important?"

Several thousand men and women from all parts of the United States and Canada have listened to these questions and worked through the answers with me in a session I have called "Developing A Career and Life Stategy." A significant part of the session is involved with managing stress. In New York, San Francisco, Los Angeles, Chicago, Dallas, Atlanta, Toronto and other cities I have seen the same response. "I want to know more about dealing with stress. I want to know more about myself." That is why it is important for us to consider Type C behavior as well as A and B behavior, and that makes us think of another physician.

Dr. Selye's prescription from the Bible—earn thy neighbor's love—is drawn from a statement that Christ made in the twenty-second chapter of Matthew. Earlier in the same chapter Jesus had responded to a teacher of religious law who tried to trap him. "Teacher," he asked, "which is the greatest commandment in the Law?" Jesus answered, "You must love the Lord your God with all your heart, with all your soul, and with all your mind. This is the greatest and most important commandment. The second most important commandment is like it: You must love your fellowman [neighbor] as yourself" (TEV).

In today's stressful times, the whole law of God and the whole law of ultimate health as well, still depends on these two commandments given by Jesus as a physician as well as a teacher. What Drs. Maslow and Selye, and others such as Drs. Freidman and Rosenman have prepared the way for (though they seem not to have realized it) is our ultimate realization that there is a way of inner purpose, achievement and peace that is distinct from A or B. These men seem to have sensed that there is a need for *something* more and have even prescribed some steps to get there—each in his own way. But the way Jesus defined is through self-abandonment rather than self-actualization or becoming a B type. We will call this abandonment Type C behavior. It was not only presented by its chief advocate, Jesus Christ, it was *lived* by him for 33 years. Type C behavior has both eustress and distress. It is as real as A or B but cannot be acquired in the same way. It is elusive even to people who have become Christians. So we need to take another look at Type C behavior in terms of stressful living.

TYPE C

Type C people are committed not just to something but to *someone* outside themselves. They do not have as their central purpose the expanding of self or the elimination of stress or even the constant attempt to live up to their Christian commitment. That is stressful living in itself. Instead, they have literally denied themselves, not only in favor of a life attitude of service to a relationship they believe in, but they have even *denied their own way* of doing it. They consider that the strongest motivation in life is *not* living up to their ego ideal—as powerful as that has become in our world—but of serving as an empty channel of wisdom, strength and love. They don't try harder. They yield more. The more they yield, the more they accomplish, and the more freedom from stressful living they have.

The response made by Jesus to the Law teacher is of deep importance, not only because Jesus boldly stated what the greatest commandment was, but because he defined the precise order in which we become a C person, and the specific way to do it. The secret is love and the channels or instruments of love are our (1) heart, (2) soul and (3) mind, *in that order.* Jesus let us know that the way to do that is impossible without relationship. That last statement is the rock-solid foundation of the Type C person. The Apostle Peter discovered that very quickly and articulated it later on in his first book, where he spoke of the "impossible road," meaning that we can't find our way alone. Today, when we look at the two commandments of Jesus, we know down inside it is impossible to love God with all our hearts and souls and minds. Maybe *some* portion of our heart, but not all. We know we need some very powerful help and even then we can miss. That is why Jesus said the words to those who stayed around long enough to hear, "If anyone wants to come with me, he must forget himself . . . For whoever wants to save his own life will lose it; but whoever loses his life for my sake will find it." (Matthew 16:24,25 TEV). This is exactly opposite from the hard-charging Type A person and different from the Type B as well. Both of them are wrapped up in themselves. They are looking for their ego ideal or self-actualization, as Abraham Maslow calls it. It is different, too, from the self-sufficient Eastern meditation approach.

The Type C approach is the loving neighbor approach. It is not earning someone's love, as Dr. Selye suggests, but loving God first. But how do we love God with all we have? By getting out of the way and letting God come in to do the thing that it is impossible for us to do. The Type C person has no identity crisis. He is living, literally, out of his mind. But that's good, not alarming. Type C people aren't doing their own thing. They aren't even doing God's thing! They are letting God do God's thing in them, as lovingly as they know how. That doesn't mean they are perfect. Just as there are no perfect Type B people or A people, there are no perfect C people. But there are some who are much closer to God's perfect will than others.

Now that we have defined A, B, and C styles of life the question is which one are we in our real everyday lives? In practice we know that some people are trying to be one thing while they are really another. There are combinations of styles rather than perfect styles. There are AB people and AC people and BC people. Some are so close to A types that you'd think that's all they are. Some are so close to C types, that you'd think they are pure C's, in all their beauty and simplicity. But on some days they aren't. Some swing like pendulums, back and forth, A to B to C to A. But the models of life are clear. There is an A model who is on a wild chase, racing against time to find out who he is. And there is a B person who is not racing at all but content with who he is, regardless of his state of goodness or apathy. And there was a C person who came and served and loved unreservedly and said, "This is the way."

This C approach touches the deepest motivation there is: to find God, to serve him and to enjoy him. This is the exciting revelation to stressful people: the key to freedom from stressful living is not simply in a series of remedies, as helpful as they are. The key is heart attitude, not just mental control, something that allows real relationship to exist. If loss of relationship is a prime cause of stress then discovery of relationship is a cure. That's where Christianity comes in.

After all is considered, Christianity is not a philosophy we adopt; it is not some theory that we are loyal to; it is not some well-thought creed; it is not something that is analyzed into existence. It is a personal response—a relationship—to a heart physician named Jesus Christ. It is a commitment and love that men and women give because their hearts will no longer allow them to do anything else. It is a heart attitude.

It is the living of this heart allegiance in very freeing ways that this book is about. That is why we need to take a closer look at our hearts and decide on the approach to life that we really want. The Christian response to stress is knowing that we are not alone and then living in that knowledge in very practical ways. He is here in the middle of our pressure points. We can accept any stress that comes and respond to it, not as Christ would, but as Christ within us responds for us.

"Strange as it seems, we Christians actually do have within us a portion of the very thoughts and mind of Christ " (1 Corinthians 2:16 LB).

We receive this Christian life by personal response to Christ's offer in Revelations 3:20: "Here I am! I stand at the door and knock. If anyone hears my voice and opens the door, I will go in" (NIV).

We can become a new creature by opening the door of our heart right now, before putting this book down, and saying, "Come in, Lord Jesus."

HERE IS A GENERAL VIEW
OF SOME DIFFERENCES IN
A, B, AND C LIFE STYLES

A

- Excessive Ambition
- Driving Aggression (Achievement Oriented)
- Marked Impatience; Obsession with Time
- Dissatisfaction with Self

B

- Relaxed, Easy Going
- Pleasure Oriented
- Accepting of Life Circumstances, Not Time Oriented
- Satisfaction with Self

C

- Committed to Personal Relationship
- Service Oriented
- Life-Yielding, "Open-Channel" Attitude
- Abandonment to God